The Super Delicious Sirt Diet Cookbook

More than 100 Recipes to Lose Weight like a Celebrity!

By Lola White

Sirt Diet Recipes
for Breakfast

by Lola White

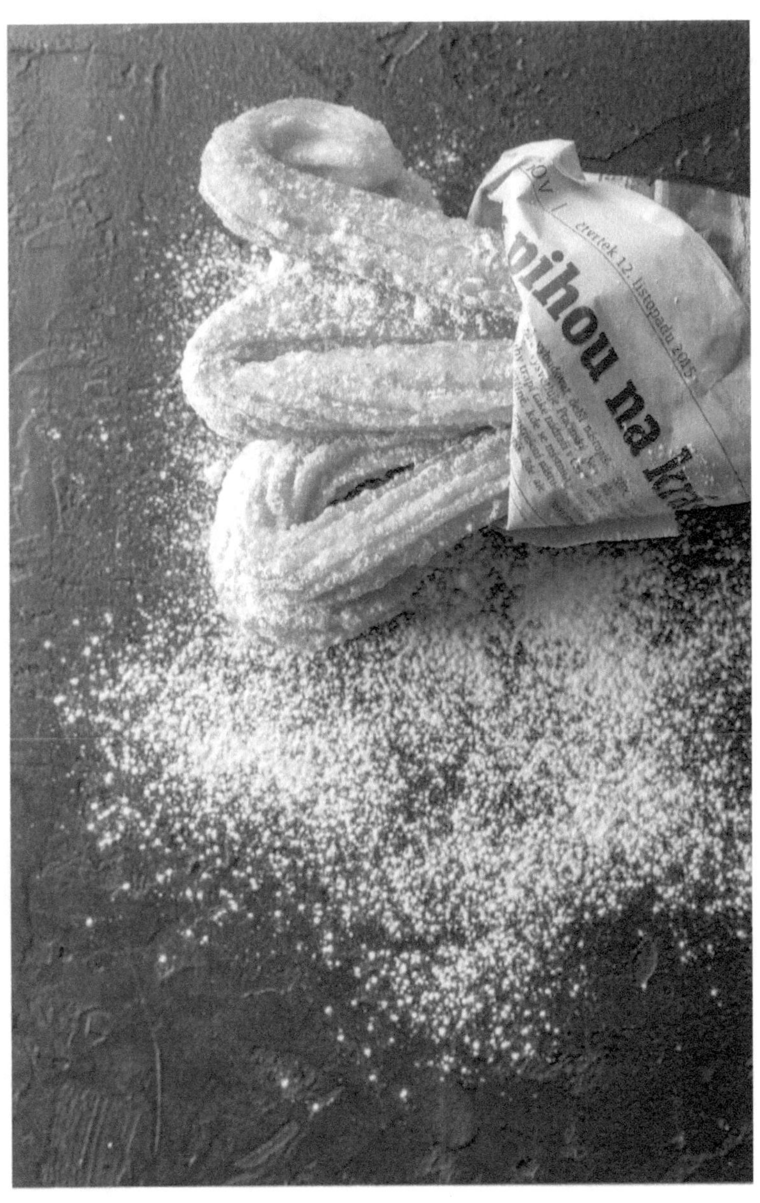

čtvrtek 12. listopadu 2015
oihou na kr

The following Book is reproduced below with the goal of providing information that is as accurate and reliable as possible. Regardless, purchasing this Book can be seen as consent to the fact that both the publisher and the author of this book are in no way experts on the topics discussed within and that any recommendations or suggestions that are made herein are for entertainment purposes only. Professionals should be consulted as needed prior to undertaking any of the action endorsed herein. This declaration is deemed fair and valid by both the American Bar Association and the Committee of Publishers Association and is legally binding throughout the United States. Furthermore, the transmission, duplication, or reproduction of any of the following work including specific information will be considered an illegal act irrespective of if it is done electronically or in print. This extends to creating a secondary or tertiary copy of the work or a recorded copy and is only allowed with the express written consent from the Publisher. All additional rights reserved. The information in the following pages is broadly considered a truthful and accurate account of facts and as such, any inattention, use, or misuse of the information in question by the reader will render any resulting actions solely under their purview. There are no scenarios in which the publisher or the original author of this work can be in any fashion deemed liable for any hardship or damages that may befall them after undertaking information described herein.

Additionally, the information in the following pages is intended only for informational purposes and should thus be thought of as universal. As befitting its nature, it is presented without assurance regarding its prolonged validity or interim quality. Trademarks that are mentioned are done without written consent and can in no way be considered an endorsement from the trademark holder.

Table of Contents

Matcha Green Juice

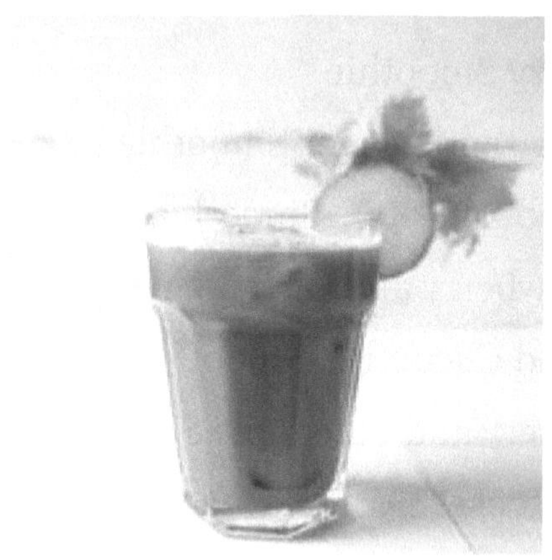

Preparation time: 10 minutes

Cooking time: 0 minutes

Servings: 2

Ingredients:

- 5 ounces fresh kale
- 2 ounces fresh arugula
- ¼ cup fresh parsley
- 4 celery stalks
- 1 green apple, cored and chopped
- 1 (1-inch) piece fresh ginger, peeled
- 1 lemon, peeled
- ½ teaspoon matcha green tea

Directions:

- Add all ingredients into a juicer and extract the juice according to the manufacturer's method.
- Pour into 2 glasses and serve immediately.

Nutrition:

- Calories: 113
- Fat: 0.6 g
- Carbohydrates: 26.71 g
- Protein: 3.8 g

Celery Juice

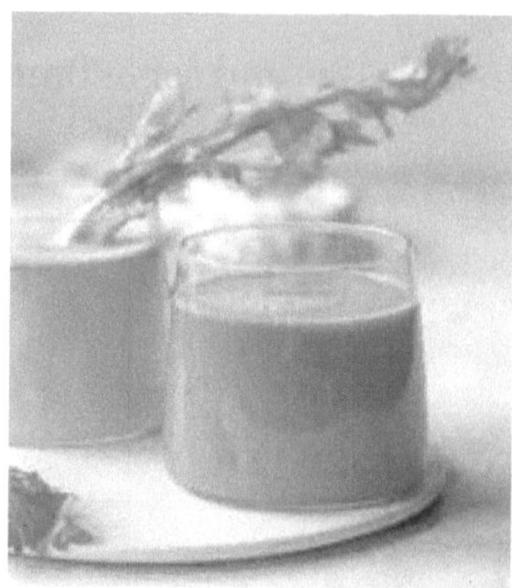

Preparation time: 10 minutes

Cooking time: 0 minutes

Servings: 2

Ingredients:

- 8 celery stalks with leaves
- 2 tablespoons fresh ginger, peeled
- 1 lemon, peeled
- ½ cup filtered water
- Pinch of salt

Directions:

- Place all the ingredients in a blender and pulse until well combined.
- Through a fine mesh strainer, strain the juice and transfer into 2 glasses.
- Serve immediately.

Nutrition:

- Calories: 32
- Fat: 0.5 g
- Carbohydrates: 6.5 g
- Protein: 1 g

Kale & Orange Juice

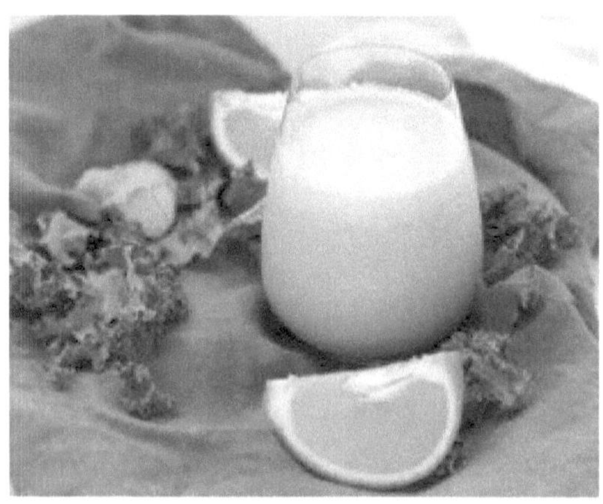

Preparation time: 10 minutes

Cooking time: 0 minutes

Servings: 2

Ingredients:

- 5 large oranges, peeled and sectioned
- 2 bunches fresh kale

Directions:

- Add all ingredients into a juicer and extract the juice according to the manufacturer's method.
- Pour into 2 glasses and serve immediately.

Nutrition:

- Calories: 315
- Fat: 0.6 g
- Carbohydrates: 75.1 g
- Protein: 10.3 g

Apple & Cucumber Juice

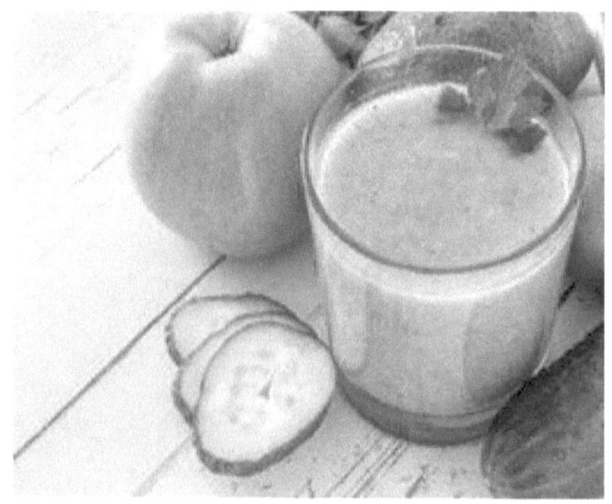

Preparation time: 10 minutes

Cooking time: 0 minutes

Servings: 2

Ingredients:

- 3 large apples, cored and sliced
- 2 large cucumbers, sliced
- 4 celery stalks
- 1 (1-inch) piece fresh ginger, peeled
- 1 lemon, peeled

Directions:

- Add all ingredients into a juicer and extract the juice according to the manufacturer's method.
- Pour into 2 glasses and serve immediately.

Nutrition:

- Calories: 230
- Fat: 1.1 g
- Carbohydrates: 59.5 g
- Protein: 3.3 g

Lemony Green Juice

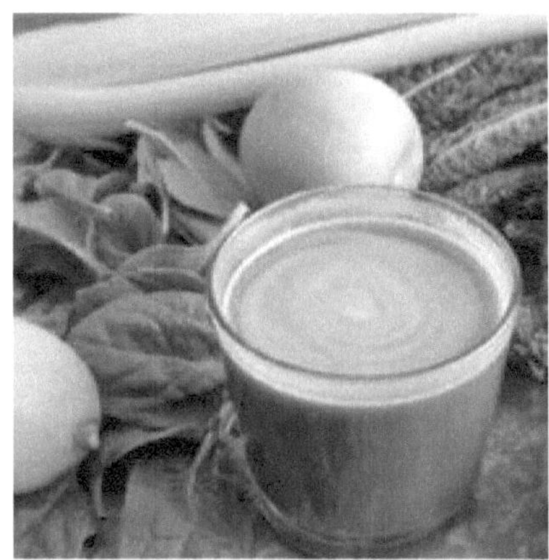

Preparation time: 10 minutes

Cooking time: 0 minutes

Servings: 2

Ingredients:

- 2 large green apples, cored and sliced
- 4 cups fresh kale leaves
- 4 tablespoons fresh parsley leaves
- 1 tablespoon fresh ginger, peeled
- 1 lemon, peeled
- ½ cup filtered water
- Pinch of salt

Directions:

- Place all the ingredients in a blender and pulse until well combined.
- Through a fine mesh strainer, strain the juice and transfer into 2 glasses.
- Serve immediately.

Nutrition:

- Calories: 196
- Fat: 0.6 g
- Carbohydrates: 47.9 g
- Protein: 5.2 g

Kale Scramble

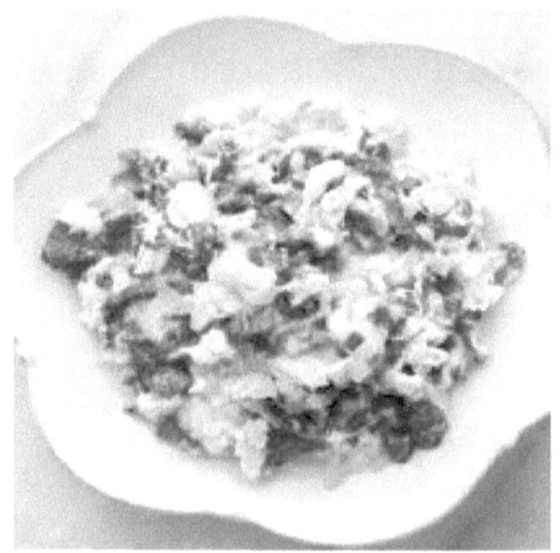

Preparation time: 10 minutes

Cooking time: 6 minutes

Servings: 2

Ingredients:

- 4 eggs
- 1/8 teaspoon ground turmeric
- Salt and ground black pepper, to taste
- 1 tablespoon water
- 2 teaspoons olive oil
- 1 cup fresh kale, tough ribs removed and chopped

Directions:

- In a bowl, add the eggs, turmeric, salt, black pepper, and water and with a whisk, beat until foamy.
- In a wok, heat the oil over medium heat.
- Add the egg mixture and stir to combine.
- Immediately, reduce the heat to medium-low and cook for about 1–2 minutes, stirring frequently.
- Stir in the kale and cook for about 3–4 minutes, stirring frequently.
- Remove from the heat and serve immediately.

Nutrition:

- Calories: 183
- Fat: 13.4 g
- Carbohydrates: 4.3 g
- Protein: 12.1 g

Buckwheat Porridge

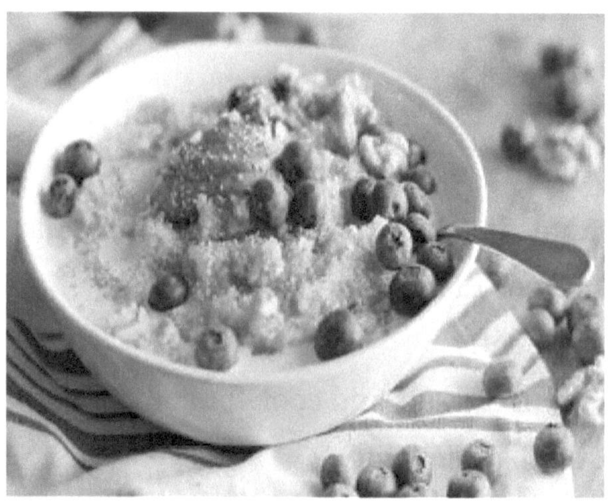

Preparation time: 10 minutes

Cooking time: 15 minutes

Servings: 2

Ingredients:

- 1 cup buckwheat, rinsed
- 1 cup unsweetened almond milk
- 1 cup water
- ½ teaspoon ground cinnamon
- ½ teaspoon vanilla extract
- 1–2 tablespoons raw honey
- ¼ cup fresh blueberries

Directions:

- In a pan, add all the ingredients (except honey and blueberries) over medium-high heat and bring to a boil.
- Now, reduce the heat to low and simmer, covered for about 10 minutes.
- Stir in the honey and remove from the heat.
- Set aside, covered, for about 5 minutes.
- With a fork, fluff the mixture, and transfer into serving bowls.
- Top with blueberries and serve.

Nutrition:

- Calories: 358
- Fat: 4.7 g
- Carbohydrates: 3.7 g
- Protein: 12 g

Blueberry Muffins

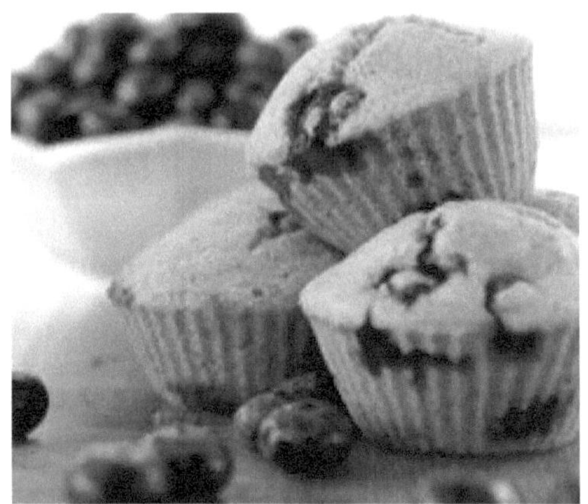

Preparation time: 15 minutes

Cooking time: 20 minutes

Servings: 8

Ingredients

- 1 cup buckwheat flour
- ¼ cup arrowroot starch
- 1½ teaspoons baking powder
- ¼ teaspoon sea salt
- 2 eggs
- ½ cup unsweetened almond milk
- 2–3 tablespoons maple syrup
- 2 tablespoons coconut oil, melted
- 1 cup fresh blueberries

Directions:

- Preheat your oven to 350°F and line 8 cups of a muffin tin.
- In a bowl, place the buckwheat flour, arrowroot starch, baking powder, and salt, and mix well.
- In a separate bowl, place the eggs, almond milk, maple syrup, and coconut oil, and beat until well combined.
- Now, place the flour mixture and mix until just combined.
- Gently, fold in the blueberries.
- Transfer the mixture into prepared muffin cups evenly.
- Bake for about 25 minutes or until a toothpick inserted in the center comes out clean.
- Remove the muffin tin from oven and place onto a wire rack to cool for about 10 minutes.
- Carefully invert the muffins onto the wire rack to cool completely before serving.

Nutrition:

- Calories: 136
- Fat: 5.3 g
- Carbohydrates: 20.7 g
- Protein: 3.5 g

Chocolate Waffles

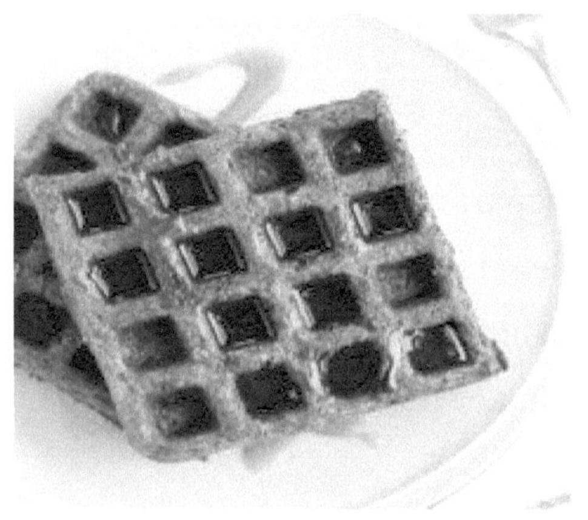

Preparation time: 15 minutes

Cooking time: 24 minutes

Servings: 8

Ingredients

- 2 cups unsweetened almond milk
- 1 tablespoon fresh lemon juice
- 1 cup buckwheat flour
- ½ cup cacao powder
- ¼ cup flaxseed meal
- 1 teaspoon baking soda

- 1 teaspoon baking powder
- ¼ teaspoons kosher salt
- 2 large eggs
- ½ cup coconut oil, melted
- ¼ cup dark brown sugar
- 2 teaspoons vanilla extract
- 2 ounces unsweetened dark chocolate, chopped roughly

Directions:

- In a bowl, add the almond milk and lemon juice and mix well.
- Set aside for about 10 minutes.
- In a bowl, place buckwheat flour, cacao powder, flaxseed meal, baking soda, baking powder, and salt, and mix well.
- In the bowl of almond milk mixture, place the eggs, coconut oil, brown sugar, and vanilla extract, and beat until smooth.
- Now, place the flour mixture and beat until smooth.
- Gently, fold in the chocolate pieces.
- Preheat the waffle iron and then grease it.

- Place the desired amount of the mixture into the preheated waffle iron and cook for about 3 minutes, or until golden-brown.
- Repeat with the remaining mixture.

Nutrition:

- Calories: 295
- Fat: 22.1 g
- Carbohydrates: 1.5 g
- Protein: 6.3 g

Moroccan Spiced Eggs

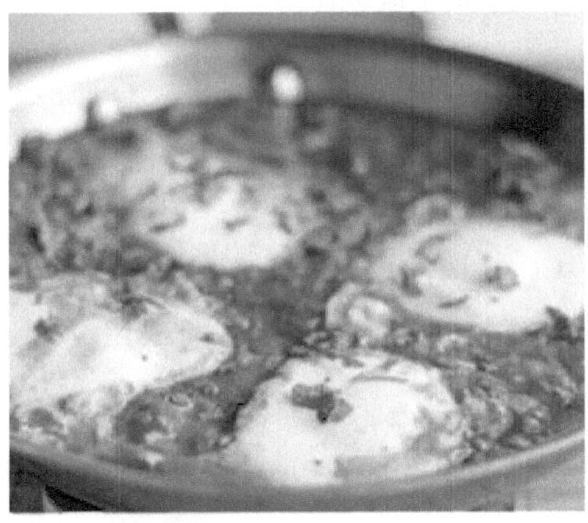

Preparation time: 1 hour

Cooking time: 50 minutes

Servings: 2

Ingredients:

- 1 tsp. olive oil
- 1 shallot, stripped and finely hacked
- 1 red (chime) pepper, deseeded and finely hacked
- 1 garlic clove, stripped and finely hacked
- 1 courgette (zucchini), stripped and finely hacked

- 1 tbsp. tomato purees (glue)
- ½ tsp. gentle stew powder
- ¼ tsp. ground cinnamon
- ¼ tsp. ground cumin
- ½ tsp. salt
- 1 × 400g (14oz) can hack tomatoes
- 1 x 400g (14oz) may chickpeas in water
- A little bunch of level leaf parsley (10g (1/3oz)), cleaved
- Four medium eggs at room temperature

Directions:

- Heat the oil in a pan; include the shallot and red (ringer) pepper and fry delicately for 5 minutes. At that point include the garlic and courgette (zucchini) and cook for one more moment or two. Include the tomato puree (glue), flavour and salt and mix through.
- Add the cleaved tomatoes and chickpeas (dousing alcohol and all) and increment the warmth to medium. With the top of the dish, stew the sauce for 30 minutes – ensure it is delicately rising all through and permit it to lessen in volume by around 33%.

- Remove from the warmth and mix in the cleaved parsley.
- Preheat the grill to 200C/180C fan/350F.
- When you are prepared to cook the eggs, bring the tomato sauce up to a delicate stew and move to a little broiler confirmation dish.
- Crack the eggs on the dish and lower them delicately into the stew. Spread with thwart and prepare in the grill for 10-15 minutes. Serve the blend in unique dishes with the eggs coasting on the top.

Nutrition:
- Calories: 116 kcal
- Protein: 6.97 g
- Fat: 5.22 g
- Carbohydrates: 13.14 g

Chilaquiles with Gochujang

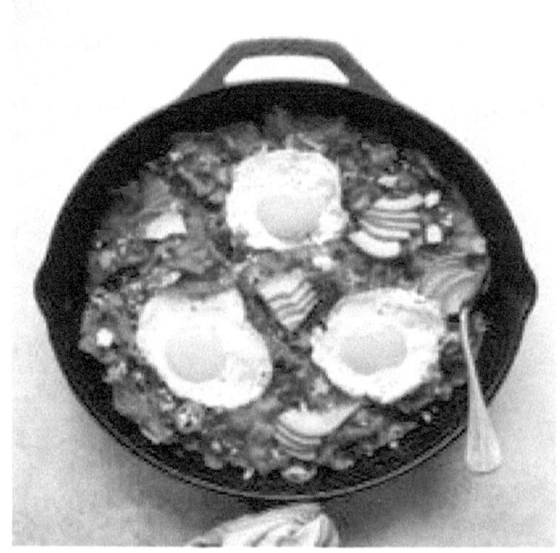

Preparation time: 30 minutes

Cooking time: 20 minutes

Servings: 2

Ingredients:

- 1 dried ancho Chile
- 2 cups of water
- 1 cup squashed tomatoes
- 2 cloves of garlic
- 1 teaspoon genuine salt

- 1/2 tablespoons Gochujang
- 5 to 6 cups tortilla chips
- 3 enormous eggs
- 1 tablespoon olive oil

Directions:

- Get the water to heat a pot. I cheated marginally and heated the water in an electric pot and emptied it into the pan.
- Add the anchor Chile to the bubbled water and drench for 15 minutes to give it an opportunity to stout up.
- When completed, use tongs or a spoon to extricate Chili. Make sure to spare the water for the sauce.
- Mix the doused Chili, 1 cup of saved high temp water, squashed tomatoes, garlic, salt and gochujang.
- Empty sauce into a large dish and heat 4 to 5 minutes. Heat and include the tortilla chips.
- Mix the chips to cover with the sauce. In a different skillet, shower a teaspoon of oil and fry an egg on top, until the whites have settled.

- Plate the egg and cook the remainder of the eggs. Sear the eggs while you heat the red sauce.
- Top the chips with the seared eggs, cotija, hacked cilantro, jalapeños, onions and avocado. Serve right away.

Nutrition:
- Calories: 484 kcal
- Protein: 14.55 g
- Fat: 18.62 g
- Carbohydrates: 64.04 g

Twice Baked Breakfast Potatoes

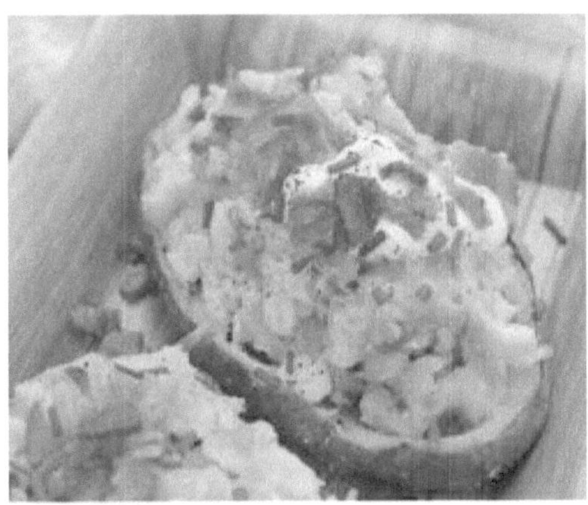

Preparation time: 1 hour 10 minutes

Cooking time: 1 hour

Servings: 2

Ingredients:

- 2 medium reddish brown potatoes, cleaned and pricked with a fork everywhere
- 2 tablespoons unsalted spread
- 3 tablespoons overwhelming cream
- 4 rashers cooked bacon
- 4 huge eggs

- ½ cup destroyed cheddar
- Daintily cut chives
- Salt and pepper to taste

Directions:

- Preheat grill to 400°F.
- Spot potatoes straightforwardly on stove rack in the focal point of the grill and prepare for 30 to 45 min.
- Evacuate and permit potatoes to cool for around 15 minutes.
- Cut every potato down the middle longwise and burrow every half out, scooping the potato substance into a blending bowl.
- Gather margarine and cream to the potato and pound into a single unit until smooth — season with salt and pepper and mix.
- Spread a portion of the potato blend into the base of each emptied potato skin and sprinkle with one tablespoon cheddar (you may make them remain pounded potato left to snack on).
- Add bacon to every half and top with a raw egg.
- Spot potatoes onto a heating sheet and come back to the appliance.

- Lower broiler temperature to 375°F and heat potatoes until egg whites simply set and yolks are as yet runny.
- Top every potato with a sprinkle of the rest of the cheddar, season with salt and pepper and finish with cut chives.

Nutrition:

- Calories: 647 kcal
- Protein: 30.46 g
- Fat: 55.79 g
- Carbohydrates: 7.45 g

Sirt Muesli

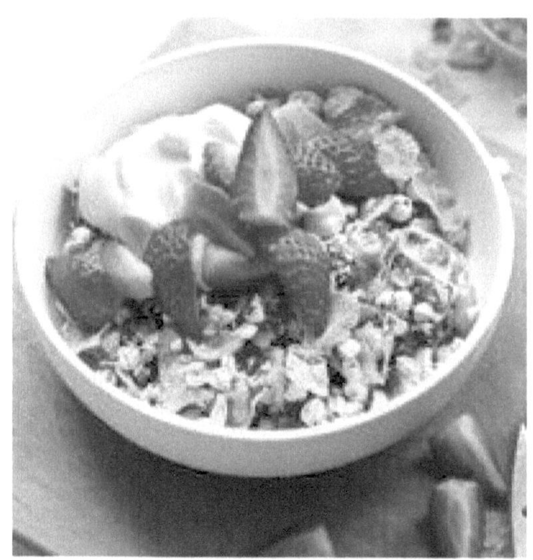

Preparation time: 30 minutes

Cooking time: 0 minutes

Servings: 2

Ingredients:

- 20g buckwheat drops
- 10g buckwheat puffs
- 15g coconut drops or dried up coconut
- 40g Medjool dates, hollowed and slashed

- 15g pecans, slashed
- 10g cocoa nibs
- 100g strawberries, hulled and slashed
- 100g plain Greek yoghurt (or vegetarian elective, for example, soya or coconut yoghurt)

Directions:

- Blend all the ingredients then put strawberries and yoghurt.
- Serve immediately.

Nutrition:

- Calories: 334 kcal
- Protein: 4.39 g
- Fat: 22.58 g
- Carbohydrates: 34.35 g

Spiced Scramble

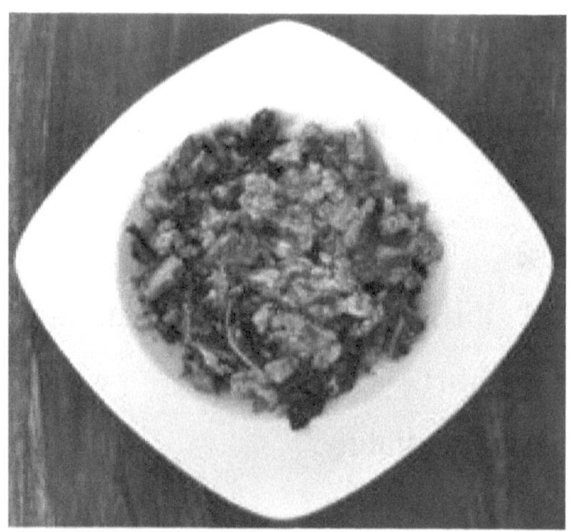

Preparation time: 5 minutes

Cooking time: 5 minutes

Servings: 1

Ingredients:

- 25g (1oz) kale, finely chopped
- 2 eggs
- 1 spring onion (scallion) finely chopped
- 1 teaspoon turmeric
- 1 tablespoon olive oil
- Sea salt
- Freshly ground black pepper

Directions:

- Crack the eggs into a bowl. Add the turmeric and whisk them and season with salt and pepper.
- Heat the oil in a frying pan, add the kale and spring onions (scallions) and cook until it has wilted.
- Pour in the beaten eggs and stir until eggs have scrambled together with the kale.

Nutrition:

- Calories: 218
- Total Fat: 15.3 g
- Cholesterol: 386.9 mg
- Sodium: 656.2 mg
- Potassium: 243.0 mg
- Carbohydrates: 2.8 g
- Protein: 17.4 g

Cheesy Baked Eggs

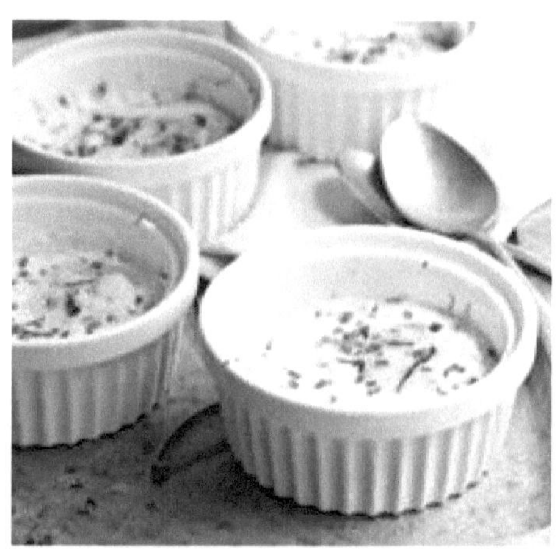

Preparation time: 5 minutes

Cooking time: 15 minutes

Servings: 4

Ingredients:

- 4 large eggs
- 75g (3oz) cheese, grated
- 25g (1oz) fresh rocket (arugula) leaves, finely chopped
- 1 tablespoon parsley
- ½ teaspoon ground turmeric
- 1 tablespoon olive oil

Directions:

- Grease each ramekin dish with a little olive oil. Divide the rocket (arugula) between the ramekin dishes then break an egg into each one.
- Sprinkle a little parsley and turmeric on top then sprinkle on the cheese.
- Place the ramekins in a preheated oven at 220C/425F for 15 minutes, until the eggs are set and the cheese is bubbling.

Nutrition:

- Calories: 67
- Total Fat: 4 g
- Cholesterol: 12 mg
- Sodium: 265 mg
- Potassium: 84 mg
- Total Carbohydrates: 0.2 g
- Protein: 8 g

Chilled Strawberry and Walnut Porridge

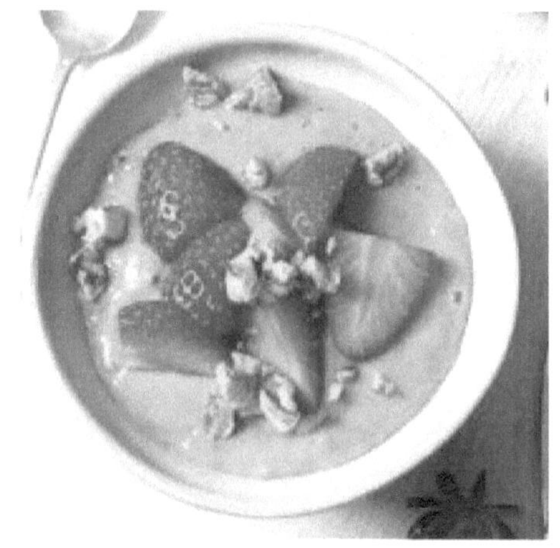

Preparation time: 10 minutes

Cooking time: 12 hours

Servings: 1

Ingredients:

- 100g (3½ oz) strawberries
- 50g (2oz) rolled oats
- 4 walnut halves, chopped
- 1 teaspoon chia seeds
- 200mls (7fl oz) unsweetened soya milk
- 100ml (3½ oz) water

Directions:

- Place the strawberries, oats, soya milk and water into a blender and process until smooth.
- Stir in the chia seeds and mix well.
- Chill in the fridge overnight and serve in the morning with a sprinkling of chopped walnuts. It's simple and delicious.

Nutrition:

- Calories: 242
- Total Fat: 6 g
- Cholesterol: 1.3 mg
- Sodium: 37 mg
- Potassium: 207 mg
- Carbohydrates: 45 g
- Protein: 6 g

Strawberry & Nut Granola

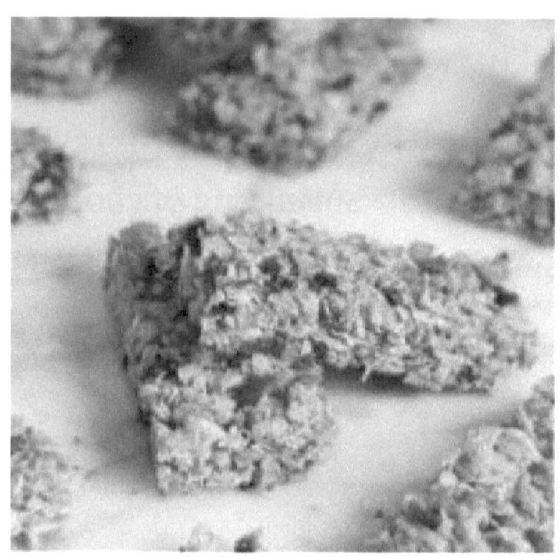

Preparation time: 10 minutes

Cooking time: 50 minutes

Servings: 12

Ingredients:

- 200g (7oz) oats
- 250g (9oz) buckwheat flakes
- 100g (3½ oz) walnuts, chopped
- 100g (3½ oz) almonds, chopped
- 100g (3½ oz) dried strawberries
- 1½ teaspoons ground ginger
- 1½ teaspoons ground cinnamon

- 120mls (4fl oz) olive oil
- 2 tablespoon honey

Directions:

- Combine the oats, buckwheat flakes, nuts, ginger and cinnamon.
- In a saucepan, warm the oil and honey. Stir until the honey has melted.
- Pour the warm oil into the dry ingredients and mix well.
- Spread the mixture out on a large baking tray (or two) and bake in the oven at 150C (300F) for around 50 minutes until the granola is golden.
- Allow it to cool. Add in the dried berries.

Nutrition:

- Calories: 220
- Fat: 3 g
- Carbohydrates: 44 g
- Protein: 6 g

Strawberry Buckwheat Pancakes

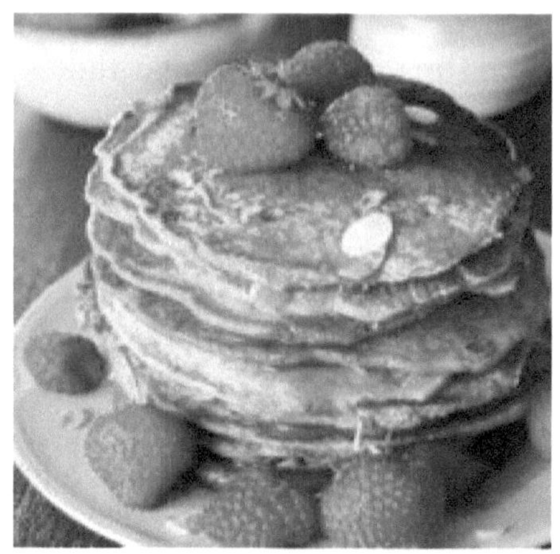

Preparation time: 10 minutes

Cooking time: 20 minutes

Servings: 4

Ingredients:

- 100g (3½oz) strawberries, chopped
- 100g (3½ oz) buckwheat flour
- 1 egg
- 250mls (8fl oz) milk
- 1 teaspoon olive oil
- 1 teaspoon olive oil for frying

- Freshly squeezed juice of 1 orange

Directions:

- Pour the milk into a bowl and mix in the egg and a teaspoon of olive oil.
- Sift in the flour to the liquid mixture until smooth and creamy.
- Allow it to rest for 15 minutes. Heat a little oil in a pan and pour in a quarter of the mixture (or to the size you prefer.)
- Sprinkle in a quarter of the strawberries into the batter.
- Cook for around 2 minutes on each side.
- Serve hot with a drizzle of orange juice.
- You could try experimenting with other berries such as blueberries and blackberries.

Nutrition:

- Calories: 76
- Fat: 3 g
- Cholesterol: 26 mg
- Sodium: 184 mg
- Potassium: 17 mg
- Carbohydrates: 4 g
- Protein: 2 g

Poached Eggs & Rocket (Arugula)

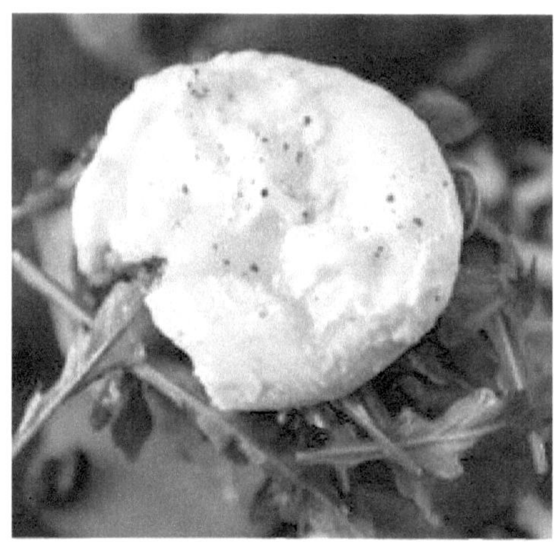

Preparation time: 3 minutes

Cooking time: 5 minutes

Servings: 2

Ingredients:

- 2 eggs
- 25g (1oz) fresh rocket (arugula)
- 1 teaspoon olive oil
- Sea salt
- Freshly ground black pepper

Directions:

- Scatter the rocket (arugula) leaves onto a plate and drizzle the olive oil over them.
- Bring a shallow pan of water to the boil, add in the eggs and cook until the whites become firm.
- Serve the eggs on top of the rocket and season with salt and pepper.

Nutrition:

- Calories: 166
- Total Fat: 10 g
- Total Carbohydrates: 7 g
- Protein: 12 g

Chocolate Berry Blend

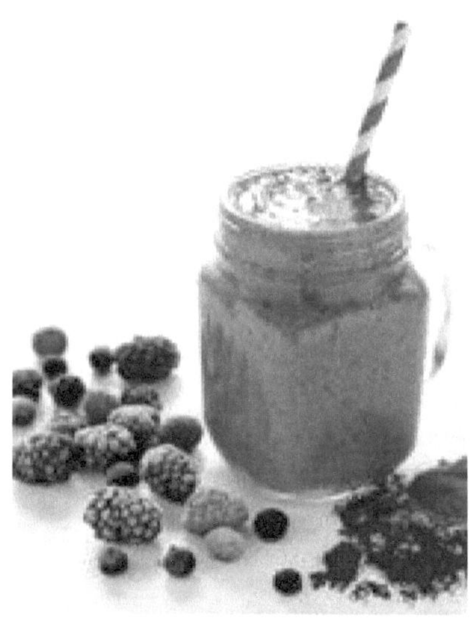

Preparation time: 5 minutes

Cooking time: 5 minutes

Servings: 1

Ingredients:

- 50g (2oz) blueberries
- 50g (2oz) strawberries
- 1 tablespoon 100% cocoa powder or cacao nibs
- 200mls (7fl oz) unsweetened soya milk

Directions:

- Place all of the ingredients into a blender with enough water to cover them and process until smooth.

Nutrition:

- Calories: 150
- Fat: 9 g
- Sodium: 30 mg
- Carbohydrates: 17 g
- Protein: 3 g
- Fiber: 2 g
- Sugar: 14 g

Mushroom & Red Onion Buckwheat Pancakes

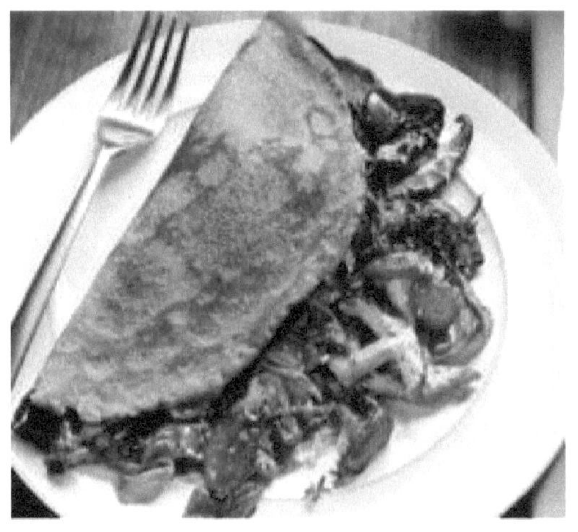

Preparation time: 5 minutes

Cooking time: 10 minutes

Servings: 2

Ingredients:

For the pancakes:

- 125g (4oz) buckwheat flour
- 1 egg
- 150mls (5fl oz) semi-skimmed milk
- 150mls (5fl oz) water
- 1 teaspoon olive oil for frying

For the filling:

- 1 red onion, chopped
- 75g (3½ oz) mushrooms, sliced
- 50g (2oz) spinach leaves
- 1 tablespoon fresh parsley, chopped
- 1 teaspoon olive oil
- 50g (2oz) rocket (arugula) leaves

Directions:

- Sift the flour into a bowl and mix in an egg.
- Pour in the milk and water and mix to a smooth batter. Set aside.
- Heat a teaspoon of olive oil in a pan. Add the onion and mushrooms and cook for 5 minutes.
- Add the spinach and allow it to wilt. Set aside and keep it warm. Heat a teaspoon of oil in a frying pan and pour in half of the batter.
- Cook for 2 minutes on each side until golden.
- Spoon the spinach and mushroom mixture onto the pancake and add the parsley.
- Fold it over and serve onto a scattering of rocket (arugula) leaves. Repeat for the remaining mixture.

Nutrition:

- Calories: 109
- Fat: 5 g
- Sodium: 61 mg
- Potassium: 339 mg
- Carbohydrates: 34 g
- Protein: 6 g

Cream of Broccoli & Kale Soup

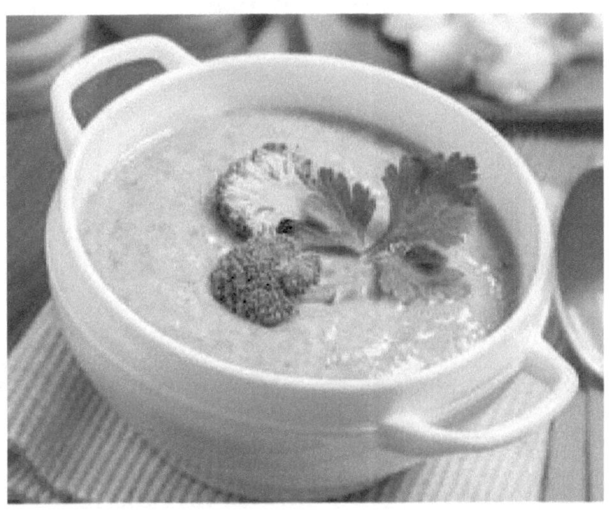

Preparation time: 10 minutes

Cooking time: 30 minutes

Servings: 4

Ingredients:

- 250g (9oz) broccoli
- 250g (9oz) kale
- 1 potato, peeled and chopped
- 1 red onion, chopped
- 600mls (1 pint) vegetable stock
- 300mls (½ pint) milk

- 1 tablespoon olive oil
- Sea salt
- Freshly ground black pepper

Directions:
- Heat the olive oil in a saucepan, add the onion and cook for 5 minutes.
- Add in the potato, kale and broccoli and cook for 5 minutes.
- Pour in the stock (broth) and milk and simmer for 20 minutes.
- Using a food processor or hand blender, process the soup until smooth and creamy.
- Season it with salt and pepper.

Nutrition:
- Calories: 123
- Total Fat: 7 g
- Cholesterol: 16 mg
- Sodium: 528 mg
- Potassium: 667 mg
- Total Carbohydrates: 13.4 g
- Protein: 5 g

French Onion Soup

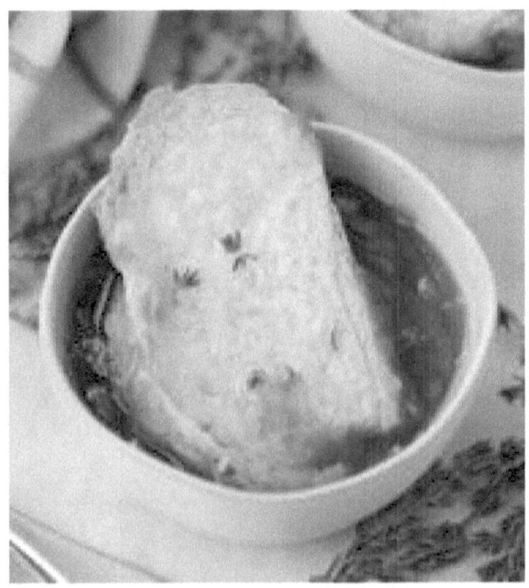

Preparation time: 10 minutes

Cooking time: 55 minutes

Servings: 4

Ingredients:

- 750g (1¾ lbs) red onions, thinly sliced
- 50g (2oz) Cheddar cheese, grated (shredded)
- 12g (½ oz) butter
- 2 teaspoons flour
- 2 slices Wholemeal bread

- 900mls (1½ pints) beef stock (broth)
- 1 tablespoon olive oil

Directions:

- Heat the butter and oil in a large pan. Add the onions and gently cook on a low heat for 25 minutes, stirring occasionally.
- Add in the flour and stir well. Pour in the stock (broth) and keep stirring.
- Bring to the boil, reduce the heat and simmer for 30 minutes.
- Cut the slices of bread into triangles, sprinkle with cheese and place them under a hot grill (broiler) until the cheese has melted.
- Serve the soup into bowls and add 2 triangles of cheesy toast on top. Enjoy.

Nutrition:

- Calories: 290
- Total Fat: 9 g
- Total Carbohydrates: 33 g
- Protein: 17 g

Cheesy Buckwheat Cakes

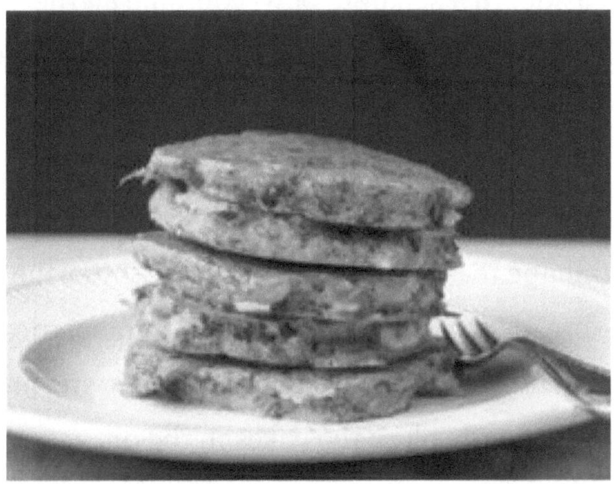

Preparation time: 4 minutes

Cooking time: 4 minutes

Servings: 2

Ingredients:

- 100g (3½oz) buckwheat, cooked and cooled
- 1 large egg
- 25g (1oz) cheddar cheese, grated (shredded)
- 25g (1oz) Wholemeal breadcrumbs
- 2 shallots, chopped
- 2 tablespoons fresh parsley, chopped
- 1 tablespoon olive oil

Directions:

- Crack the egg into a bowl, whisk it then set aside. In a separate bowl combine all the buckwheat, cheese, shallots and parsley and mix well.
- Pour in the beaten egg to the buckwheat mixture and stir well.
- Shape the mixture into patties. Scatter the breadcrumbs on a plate and roll the patties in them. Heat the olive oil in a large frying pan and gently place the cakes in the oil.
- Cook for 3-4 minutes on either side until slightly golden.

Nutrition:

- Calories: 240
- Total Fat: 4 g
- Sodium: 380 mg
- Total Carbohydrates: 40 g
- Protein: 11 g

Lentil Soup

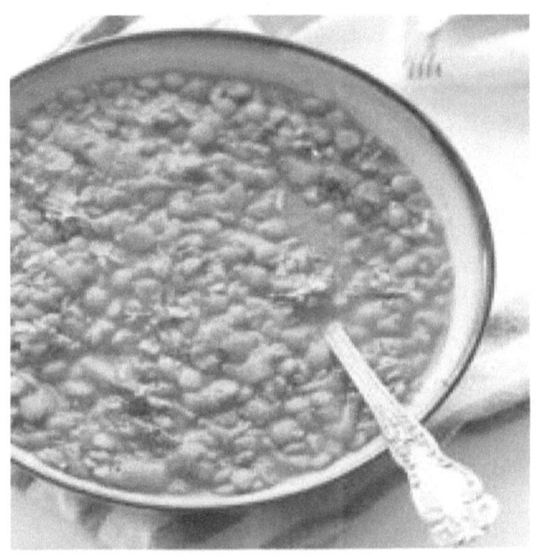

Preparation time: 5 minutes

Cooking time: 55 minutes

Servings: 4

Ingredients:

- 175g (6oz) red lentils
- 1 red onion, chopped
- 1 clove of garlic, chopped
- 2 sticks of celery, chopped
- 2 carrots, chopped
- ½ bird eye chili
- 1 teaspoon ground cumin

- 1 teaspoon ground turmeric
- 1 teaspoon ground coriander (cilantro)
- 1200mls (2 pints) vegetable stock (broth)
- 2 tablespoons olive oil
- Sea salt
- Freshly ground black pepper

Directions:

- Heat the oil in a saucepan and add the onion and cook for 5 minutes.
- Add in the carrots, lentils, celery, chili, coriander (cilantro), cumin, turmeric and garlic and cook for 5 minutes.
- Pour in the stock (broth), bring it to the boil, reduce the heat and simmer for 45 minutes.
- Using a hand blender or food processor, puree the soup until smooth.
- Season it with salt and pepper. Serve.

Nutrition:

- Calories: 194
- Total Fat: 1 g
- Sodium: 231 mg
- Total Carbohydrates: 34 g
- Protein: 13
- Fiber: 2 g

Apple Pancakes

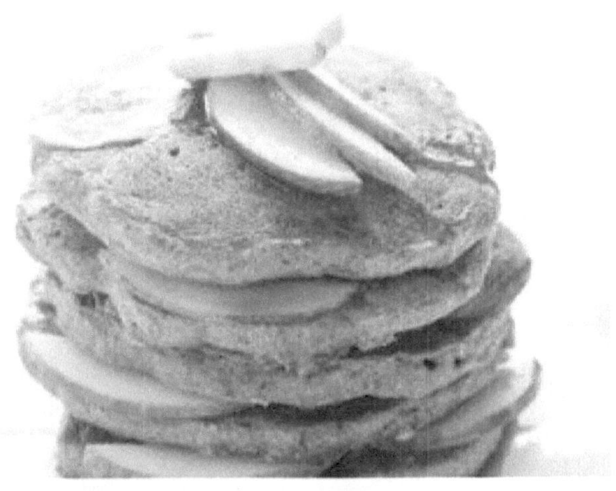

Preparation time: 15 minutes

Cooking time: 24 minutes

Servings: 6

Ingredients:

- ½ cup buckwheat flour
- 2 tablespoons coconut sugar
- 1 teaspoon baking powder
- ½ teaspoon ground cinnamon
- 1/3 cup unsweetened almond milk
- 1 egg, beaten lightly

- 2 granny smith apples, peeled, cored, and grated

Directions:

- In a bowl, place the flour, coconut sugar, and cinnamon, and mix well.
- In another bowl, place the almond milk and egg and beat until well combined.
- Now, place the flour mixture and mix until well combined.
- Fold in the grated apples.
- Heat a lightly greased non-stick wok over medium-high heat.
- Add desired amount of mixture and with a spoon, spread into an even layer.
- Cook for 1–2 minutes on each side.
- Repeat with the remaining mixture.
- Serve warm with the drizzling of honey.

Nutrition:

- Calories 93
- Total Fat 2.1 g
- Saturated Fat 1 g
- Cholesterol 27 mg

- Sodium 23 mg
- Total Carbohydrates 22 g
- Fiber 3 g
- Sugar 12.1 g
- Protein 2.5 g

Matcha Pancakes

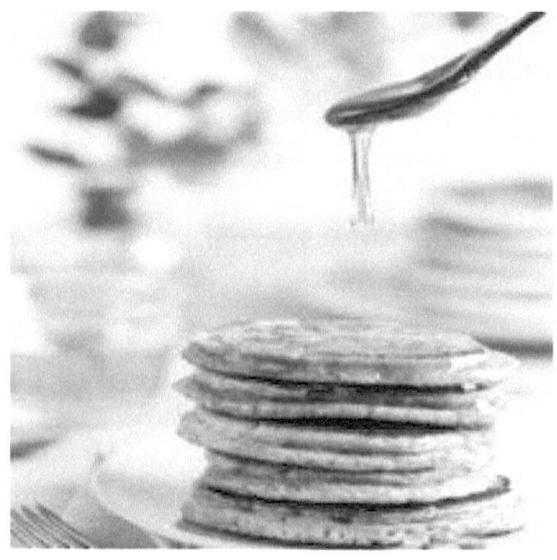

Preparation time: 15 minutes

Cooking time: 24 minutes

Servings: 6

Ingredients:

- 2 tablespoons flax meal
- 5 tablespoons warm water
- 1 cup spelt flour
- 1 cup buckwheat flour
- 1 tablespoon matcha powder
- 1 tablespoon baking powder
- Pinch of salt

- ¾ cup unsweetened almond milk
- 1 tablespoon olive oil
- 1 teaspoon vanilla extract
- 1/3 cup raw honey

Directions:

- In a bowl, add the flax meal and warm water and mix well. Set aside for about 5 minutes.
- In another bowl, place the flours, matcha powder, baking powder, and salt, and mix well.
- In the bowl of flax meal mixture, place the almond milk, oil, and vanilla extract, and beat until well combined.
- Now, place the flour mixture and mix until a smooth textured mixture is formed.
- Heat a lightly greased non-stick wok over medium-high heat.
- Add desired amount of mixture and with a spoon, spread into an even layer.
- Cook for about 2–3 minutes.
- Carefully, flip the side and cook for about 1 minute.
- Repeat with the remaining mixture.
- Serve warm with the drizzling of honey.

Nutrition:

- Calories 232
- Total Fat 4.6 g
- Saturated Fat 0.6 g
- Cholesterol 0 mg
- Sodium 56 mg
- Total Carbohydrates 46.3 g
- Fiber 5.3 g
- Sugar 16.2 g
- Protein 6 g

Chocolate Muffins

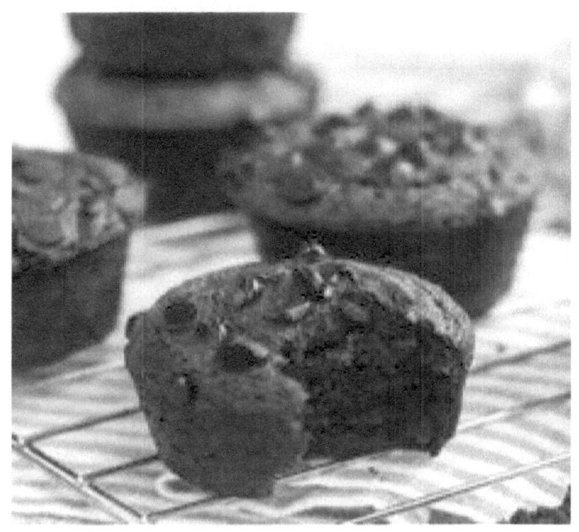

Preparation time: 15 minutes

Cooking time: 20 minutes

Servings: 6

Ingredients:

- ½ cup buckwheat flour
- ½ cup almond flour
- 4 tablespoons arrowroot powder
- 4 tablespoons cacao powder
- 1 teaspoon baking powder
- ½ teaspoon bicarbonate soda

- ½ cup boiled water
- 1/3 cup maple syrup
- 1/3 cup coconut oil, melted
- 1 tablespoon apple cider vinegar
- ½ cup unsweetened dark chocolate chips

Directions:

- Preheat your oven to 350°F. Line 6 cups of a muffin tin with paper liners.
- In a bowl, place the flours, arrowroot powder, baking powder, and bicarbonate of soda, and mix well.
- In a separate bowl, place the boiled water, maple syrup, and coconut oil, and beat until well combined.
- Now, place the flour mixture and mix until just combined.
- Gently, fold in the chocolate chips.
- Transfer the mixture into prepared muffin cups evenly.
- Bake for about 20 minutes, or until a toothpick inserted in the center comes out clean.
- Remove the muffin tin from oven and place onto a wire rack to cool for about 10 minutes.

- Carefully invert the muffins onto the wire rack to cool completely before serving.

Nutrition:

- Calories 410
- Total Fat 28.6 g
- Saturated Fat 17.8 g
- Sodium 25 mg
- Total Carbohydrates 32.5 g
- Fiber 5.8 g
- Protein 4.6 g

Kale & Mushroom Frittata

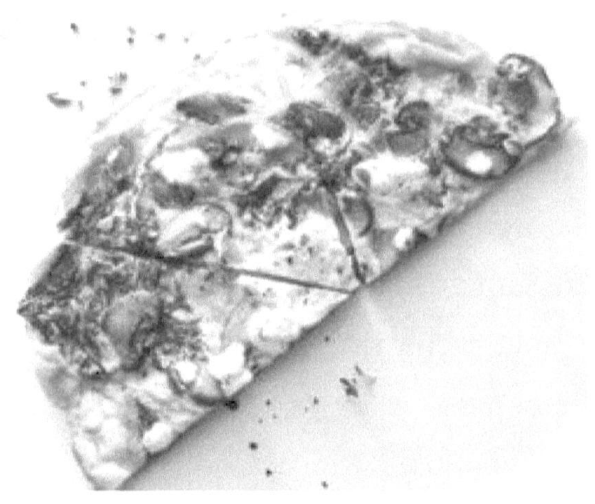

Preparation time: 15 minutes

Cooking time: 30 minutes

Servings: 5

Ingredients:

- 8 eggs
- ½ cup unsweetened almond milk
- Salt and ground black pepper, to taste
- 1 tablespoon olive oil
- 1 onion, chopped
- 1 garlic clove, minced

- 1 cup fresh mushrooms, chopped
- 1½ cups fresh kale, tough ribs removed and chopped

Directions:

- Preheat oven to 350°F.
- In a large bowl, place the eggs, coconut milk, salt, and black pepper, and beat well. Set aside.
- In a large ovenproof wok, heat the oil over medium heat and sauté the onion and garlic for about 3–4 minutes.
- Add the squash, kale, bell pepper, salt, and black pepper, and cook for about 8–10 minutes.
- Stir in the mushrooms and cook for about 3–4 minutes.
- Add the kale and cook for about 5 minutes.
- Place the egg mixture on top evenly and cook for about 4 minutes, without stirring.
- Transfer the wok in the oven and bake for about 12–15 minutes or until desired doneness.
- Remove from the oven and place the frittata side for about 3–5 minutes before serving.
- Cut into desired sized wedges and serve.

Nutrition:

- Calories 151
- Total Fat 10.2 g
- Saturated Fat 2.6 g
- Cholesterol 262 mg
- Sodium 158 mg
- Total Carbohydrates 5.6 g
- Fiber 1 g
- Sugar 1.7 g
- Protein 10.3 g

Kale, Apple, and Cranberry Salad

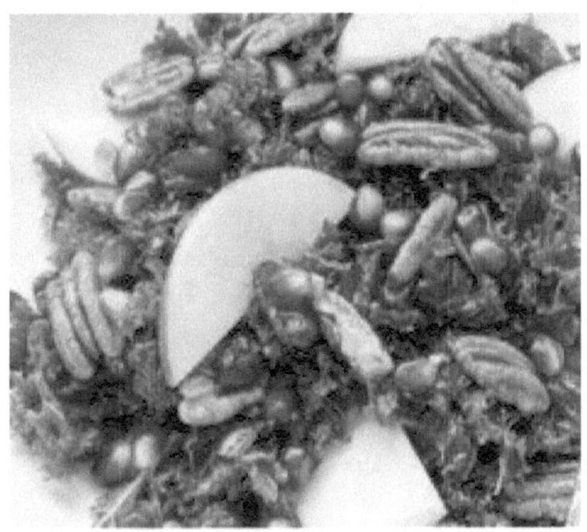

Preparation time: 10 minutes

Cooking time: 15 minutes

Servings: 4

Ingredients:

- 6 cups fresh baby kale
- 3 large apples, cored and sliced
- ¼ cup unsweetened dried cranberries
- ¼ cup almonds, sliced
- 2 tablespoons extra-virgin olive oil
- 1 tablespoon raw honey

- Salt and ground black pepper, to taste

Directions:

- In a salad bowl, place all the ingredients and toss to coat well.
- Serve immediately.

Nutrition:

- Calories 253
- Total Fat 10.3 g
- Saturated Fat 1.2 g
- Cholesterol 0 mg
- Sodium 84 mg
- Total Carbohydrates 40.7 g
- Fiber 6.6 g
- Sugar 22.7 g
- Protein 4.7 g

Sirt Diet Snacks and Desserts

By Lola White

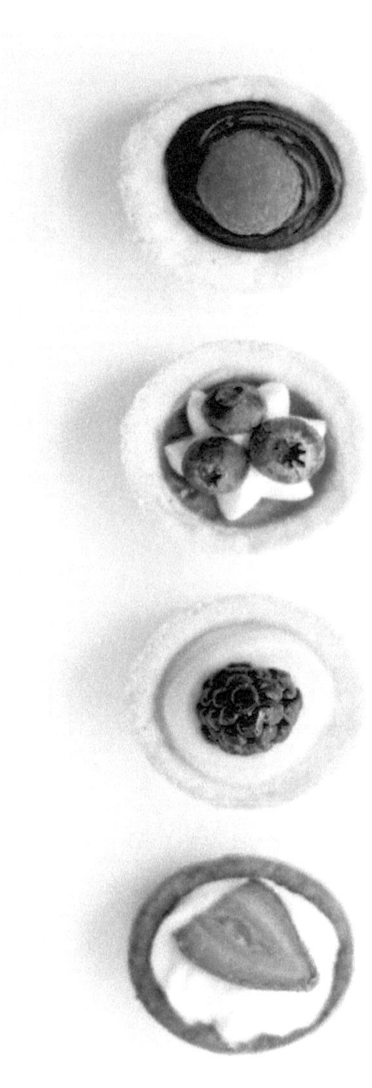

The following Book is reproduced below with the goal of providing information that is as accurate and reliable as possible. Regardless, purchasing this Book can be seen as consent to the fact that both the publisher and the author of this book are in no way experts on the topics discussed within and that any recommendations or suggestions that are made herein are for entertainment purposes only. Professionals should be consulted as needed prior to undertaking any of the action endorsed herein. This declaration is deemed fair and valid by both the American Bar Association and the Committee of Publishers Association and is legally binding throughout the United States. Furthermore, the transmission, duplication, or reproduction of any of the following work including specific information will be considered an illegal act irrespective of if it is done electronically or in print. This extends to creating a secondary or tertiary copy of the work or a recorded copy and is only allowed with the express written consent from the Publisher. All additional rights reserved. The information in the following pages is broadly considered a truthful and accurate account of facts and as such, any inattention, use, or misuse of the information in question by the reader will render any resulting actions solely under their purview. There are no scenarios in which the publisher or the original author of this work can be in any fashion deemed liable for any hardship or damages that may befall them after undertaking information described herein. Additionally, the information in the following pages is intended only for informational purposes and should thus be thought of as universal. As befitting its nature, it is presented without assurance regarding its prolonged validity or interim quality. Trademarks that are mentioned are done without written consent and can in no way be considered an endorsement from the trademark holder.

Table of Contents

Baby Spinach Snack

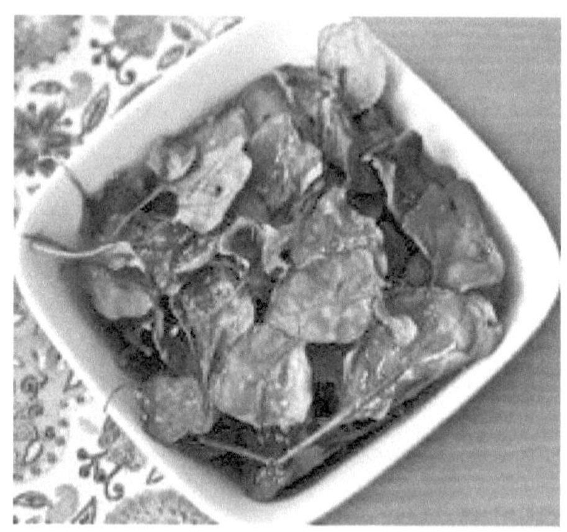

Preparation time: 10 minutes

Cooking time: 10 minutes

Servings: 1

Ingredients:

2 cups baby spinach, washed

A pinch of black pepper

½ tablespoon olive oil

½ teaspoon garlic powder

Directions:

Spread the baby spinach on a lined baking sheet, add oil, black pepper and garlic powder, toss a bit.

Bake at 350 degrees F for 10 minutes, divide into bowls and serve as a snack.

Enjoy!

Nutrition:

Calories: 125

Fat: 4 g

Fiber: 1 g

Carbohydrates: 4 g

Protein: 2 g

Sesame Dip

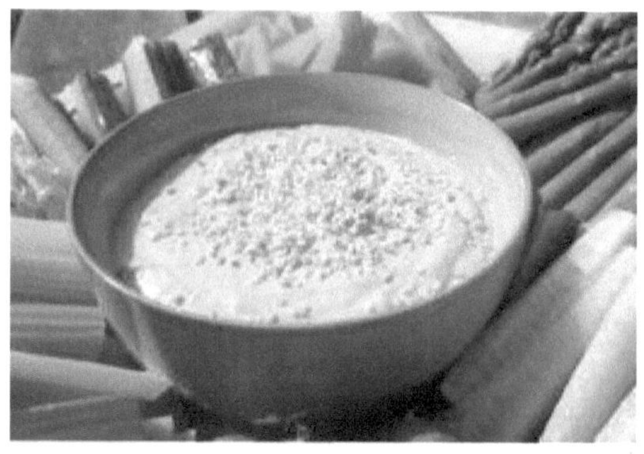

Preparation time: 10 minutes

Cooking time: 0 minutes

Servings: 1

Ingredients:

1 cup sesame seed paste, pure

Black pepper to the taste

1 cup veggie stock

½ cup lemon juice

½ teaspoon cumin, ground

3 garlic cloves, chopped

Directions:

In your food processor, mix the sesame paste with black pepper, stock, lemon juice, cumin and garlic.
Pulse very well, divide into bowls and serve as a party dip.
Enjoy!

Nutrition:

Calories: 120

Fat: 12 g

Fiber: 2 g

Carbohydrates: 7 g

Protein: 4 g

Rosemary Squash Dip

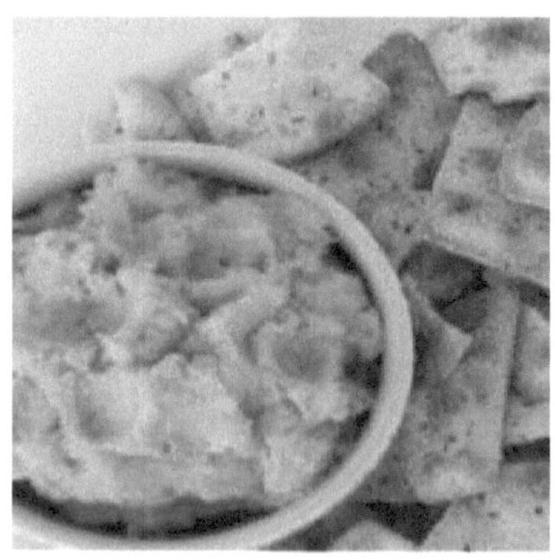

Preparation time: 10 minutes

Cooking time: 40 minutes

Servings: 1

Ingredients:

1 cup butternut squash, peeled and cubed

1 tablespoon water

Cooking spray

2 tablespoons coconut milk

2 teaspoons rosemary, dried

Black pepper to the taste

Directions:

Spread squash cubes on a lined baking sheet, spray some cooking oil, introduce in the oven, bake at 365 degrees F for 40 minutes.

Transfer to your blender, add water, milk, rosemary and black pepper, pulse well, divide into small bowls and serve. Enjoy!

Nutrition:

Calories: 182

Fat: 5 g

Fiber: 7 g

Carbohydrates: 12 g

Protein: 5 g

Bean Spread

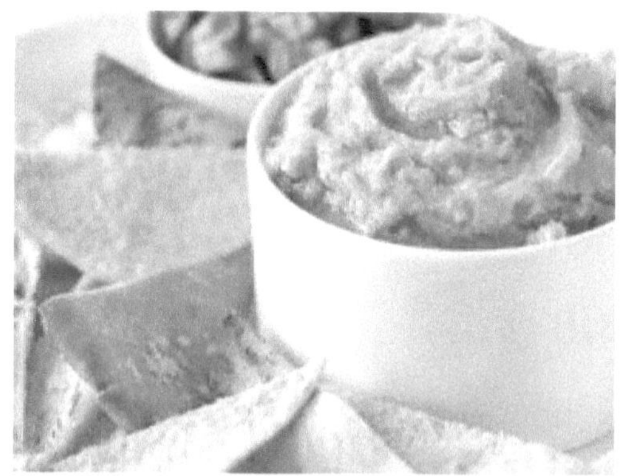

Preparation time: 10 minutes

Cooking time: 6 hours

Servings: 1

Ingredients:

1 cup white beans, dried

1 teaspoon apple cider vinegar

1 cup veggie stock

1 tablespoon water

Directions:

In your slow cooker, mix beans with stock, stir, cover, cook on Low for 6 hours.

Drain and transfer to your food processor, add vinegar and water, pulse well, divide into bowls and serve.

Enjoy!

Nutrition:

Calories: 181

Fat: 6 g

Fiber: 5 g

Carbohydrates: 9 g

Protein: 7 g

Corn Spread

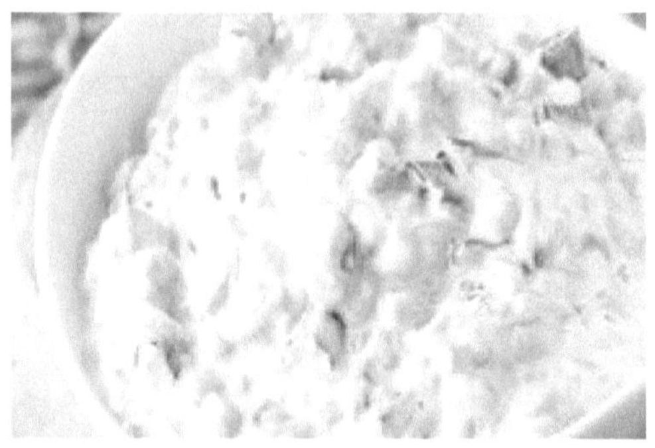

Preparation time: 10 minutes

Cooking time: 10 minutes

Servings: 1

Ingredients:

30 ounces canned corn, drained

2 green onions, chopped

½ cup coconut cream

1 jalapeno, chopped

½ teaspoon chili powder

Directions:

In a small pan, combine the corn with green onions, jalapeno and chili powder, stir, and bring to a simmer. Cook over medium heat for 10 minutes, leave aside to cool down, add coconut cream, stir well, divide into small bowls and serve as a spread.

Enjoy!

Nutrition:

Calories: 192

Fat: 5

Fiber 10

Carbohydrates: 11 g

Protein: 8 g

Mushroom Dip

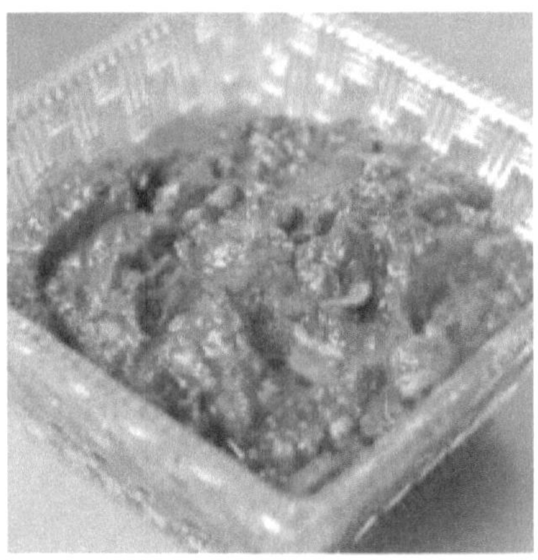

Preparation time: 10 minutes

Cooking time: 20 minutes

Servings: 1

Ingredients:

1 cup yellow onion, chopped

3 garlic cloves, minced

1 pound mushrooms, chopped

28 ounces tomato sauce, no-salt-added

Black pepper to the taste

Directions:

Put the onion in a pot, add garlic, mushrooms, black pepper and tomato sauce, and stir.

Cook over medium heat for 20 minutes, leave aside to cool down, divide into small bowls and serve.

Enjoy!

Nutrition:

Calories 215

Fat: 4 g

Fiber: 7 g

Carbohydrates: 3 g

Protein: 7 g

• Salsa Bean Dip

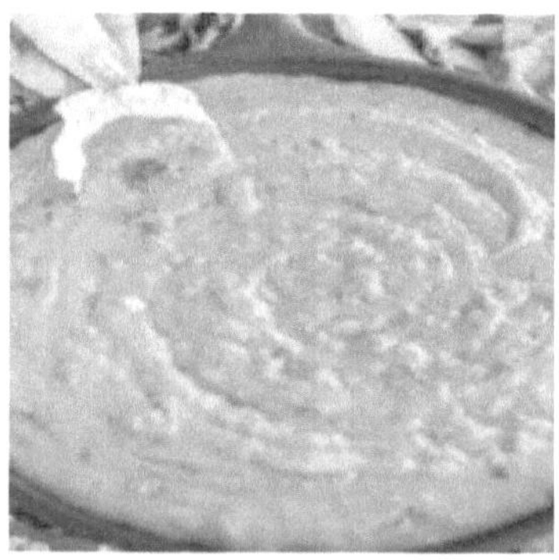

Preparation time: 10 minutes

Cooking time: 20 minutes

Servings: 1

Ingredients:

½ cup salsa

2 cups canned white beans, no-salt-added, drained and rinsed

1 cup low-fat cheddar, shredded

2 tablespoons green onions, chopped

Directions:

In a small pot, combine the beans with the green onions and salsa, stir, bring to a simmer over medium heat, and cook for 20 minutes

Add cheese, stir until it melts, and take off heat, leave aside to cool down, divide into bowls and serve.

Enjoy!

Nutrition:

Calories: 212

Fat: 5 g

Fiber: 6 g

Carbohydrates: 10 g

Protein: 8 g

Mung Beans Snack Salad

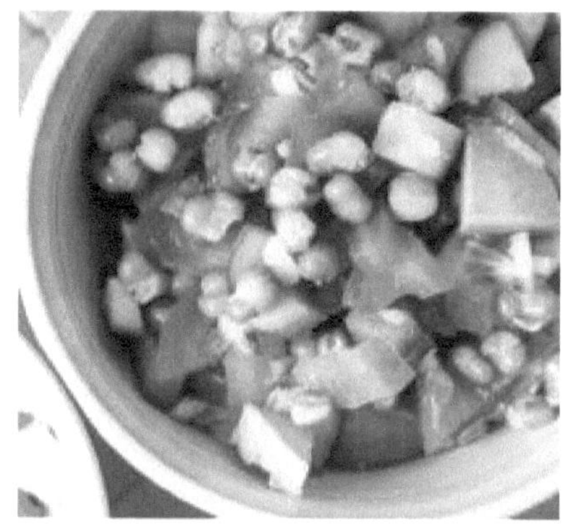

Preparation time: 10 minutes

Cooking time: 0 minutes

Servings: 1

Ingredients:

2 cups tomatoes, chopped

2 cups cucumber, chopped

3 cups mixed greens

2 cups mung beans, sprouted

2 cups clover sprouts

For the salad dressing:

1 tablespoon cumin, ground

1 cup dill, chopped

4 tablespoons lemon juice

1 avocado, pitted, peeled and roughly chopped

1 cucumber, roughly chopped

Directions:

In a salad bowl, mix tomatoes with 2 cups cucumber, greens, clover and mung sprout.

In your blender, mix cumin with dill, lemon juice, 1 cucumber and avocado, blend really well, add this to your salad, toss well and serve as a snack

Enjoy!

Nutrition:

Calories: 120

Fat: 0 g

Fiber: 2 g

Carbohydrates: 1 g

Protein: 6 g

Greek Party Dip

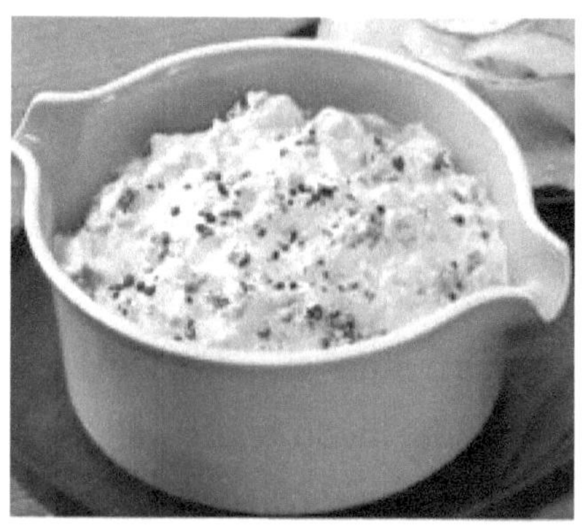

Preparation time: 10 minutes

Cooking time: 0 minutes

Servings: 1

Ingredients:

½ cup coconut cream

1 cup fat-free Greek yogurt

2 teaspoons dill, dried

2 teaspoons thyme, dried

1 teaspoon sweet paprika

2 teaspoons no-salt-added sun-dried tomatoes, chopped

2 teaspoons parsley, chopped

2 teaspoons chives, chopped

Black pepper to the taste

Directions:

In a bowl, mix cream with yogurt, dill with thyme, paprika,

tomatoes, parsley, chives and pepper, stir well.

Divide into smaller bowls and serve as a dip.

Enjoy!

Nutrition:

Calories: 100

Fat: 1 g

Fiber: 4 g

Carbohydrates: 8 g

Protein: 3 g

Zucchini Bowls

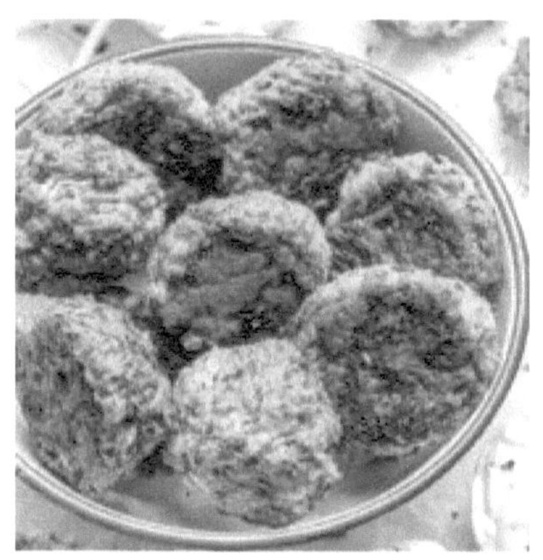

Preparation time: 10 minutes

Cooking time: 20 minutes

Servings: 12

Ingredients:

Cooking spray

½ cup dill, chopped

1 egg

½ cup whole wheat flour

Black pepper to the taste

1 yellow onion, chopped

2 garlic cloves, minced

3 zucchinis, grated

Directions:

In a bowl, mix zucchinis with garlic, onion, flour, pepper, egg and dill, stir well, shape small bowls out of this mix. Arrange them on a lined baking sheet; grease them with some cooking spray.

Bake at 400 degrees F for 20 minutes, flipping them halfway, divide them into bowls and serve as a snack. Enjoy!

Nutrition:

Calories: 120

Fat: 1 g

Fiber: 4 g

Carbohydrates: 12 g

Protein: 6 g

Baking Powder Biscuits

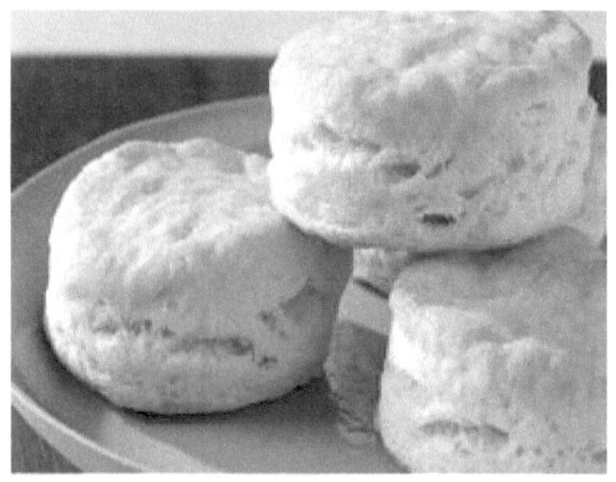

Preparation time: 10 minutes

Cooking time: 10 minutes

Servings: 1 2

Ingredients:

1 egg white

1 c. white whole-wheat flour

4 tbsp. of Non-hydrogenated vegetable shortening

1 tbsp. sugar

2/3 c. low-fat milk

1 c. unbleached all-purpose flour

4 tsps. Sodium-free baking powder

Directions:

Preheat oven to 450°F. Take out a baking sheet and set aside.

Place the flour, sugar, and baking powder into a mixing bowl and whisk well to combine.

Cut the shortening into the mixture using your fingers, and work until it resembles coarse crumbs. Add the egg white and milk and stir to combine.

Turn the dough out onto a lightly floured surface and knead 1 minute. Roll dough to ¾ inch thickness and cut into 12 rounds.

Place rounds on the baking sheet. Place baking sheet on middle rack in oven and bake 10 minutes.

Remove baking sheet and place biscuits on a wire rack to cool.

Nutrition:

Calories: 118

Fat: 4 g

Carbohydrates: 16 g

Protein: 3 g

Sugars: 0.2 g

Sodium: 294 mg

Vegan Rice Pudding

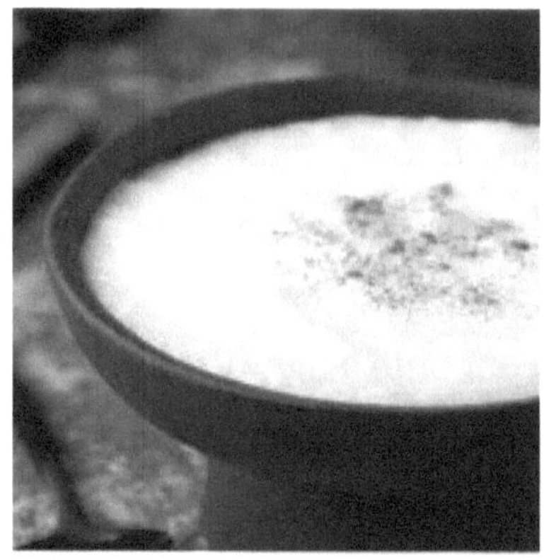

Preparation time: 5 minutes

Cooking time: 20 minutes

Servings: 8

Ingredients:

½ tsp. ground cinnamon

1 c. rinsed basmati

1/8 tsp. ground cardamom

¼ c. sugar

1/8 tsp. pure almond extract

1 quart vanilla nondairy milk

1 tsp. pure vanilla extract

Directions:

Measure all of the ingredients into a saucepan and stir well to combine. Bring to a boil over medium-high heat.

Once boiling, reduce heat to low and simmer, stirring very frequently, about 15–20 minutes.

Remove from heat and cool. Serve sprinkled with additional ground cinnamon if desired.

Nutrition:

Calories: 148

Fat: 2 g

Carbohydrates: 26 g

Protein: 4 g

Sugars: 35 g

Sodium: 150 mg

Orange and Carrots

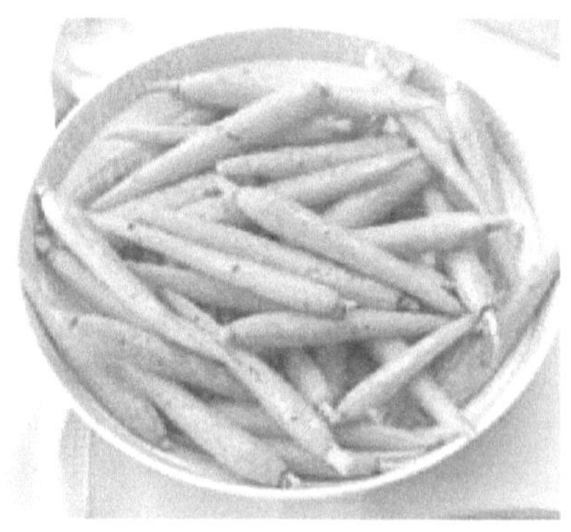

Preparation time: 5 minutes

Cooking time: 25 minutes

Servings: 1

Ingredients:

1 pound carrots, peeled and roughly sliced

1 yellow onion, chopped

1 tablespoon olive oil

Zest of 1 orange, grated

Juice of 1 orange

1 orange, peeled and cut into segments

1 tablespoon rosemary, chopped

A pinch of salt and black pepper

Directions:

Heat up a pan with the oil over medium-high heat.

Add the onion and sauté for 5 minutes.

Add the carrots, the orange zest and the other ingredients.

Cook over medium heat for 20 minutes more, divide

between plates and serve.

Nutrition:

Calories: 140

Fat: 3.9 g

Fiber: 5 g

Carbohydrates: 26.1 g

Protein: 2.1 g

Baked Broccoli and Pine Nuts

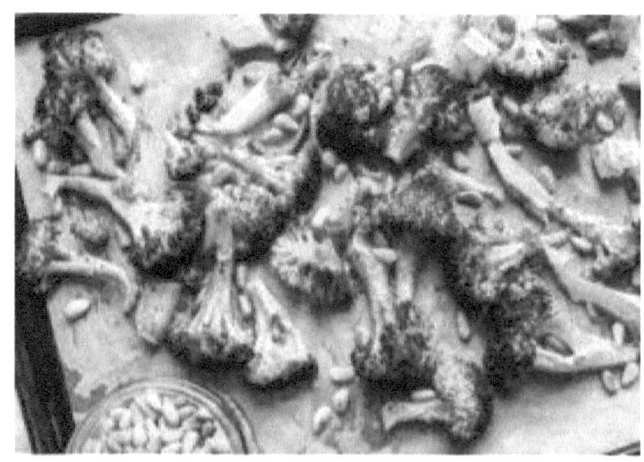

Preparation time: 10 minutes

Cooking time: 30 minutes

Servings: 1

Ingredients:

2 tablespoons olive oil

1 pound broccoli florets

1 tablespoon garlic, minced

1 tablespoon pine nuts, toasted

1 tablespoon lemon juice

2 teaspoons mustard

A pinch of salt and black pepper

Directions:

In a roasting pan, combine the broccoli with the oil, the garlic and the other ingredients, toss and bake at 380 degrees F for 30 minutes.

Divide everything between plates and serve as snack.

Nutrition:

Calories: 220

Fat: 6 g

Fiber: 2 g

Carbohydrates: 7 g

Protein: 6 g

Turmeric Carrots

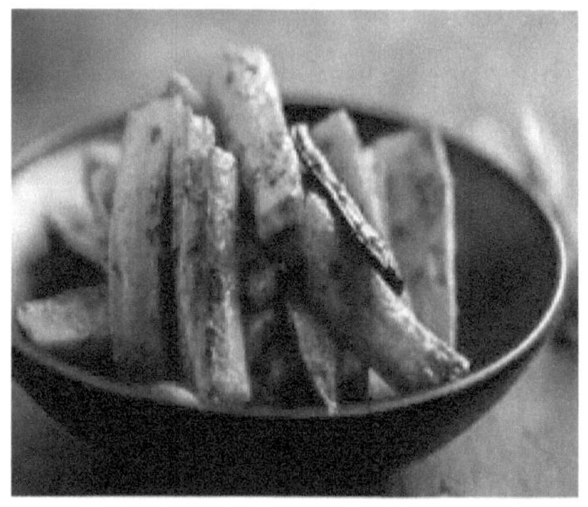

Preparation time: 10 minutes

Cooking time: 40 minutes

Servings: 1

Ingredients:

1 pound baby carrots, peeled

1 tablespoon olive oil

2 spring onions, chopped

2 tablespoons balsamic vinegar

2 garlic cloves, minced

1 teaspoon turmeric powder

1 tablespoon chives, chopped

¼ teaspoon cayenne pepper

A pinch of salt and black pepper

Directions:

Spread the carrots on a baking sheet lined with parchment paper, add the oil, the spring onions and the other ingredients, toss and bake at 380 degrees F for 40 minutes. Divide the carrots between plates and serve.

Nutrition:

Calories: 79

Fat: 3.8 g

Fiber: 3.7 g

Carbohydrates: 10.9 g

Protein: 1 g

Hawaii Salad

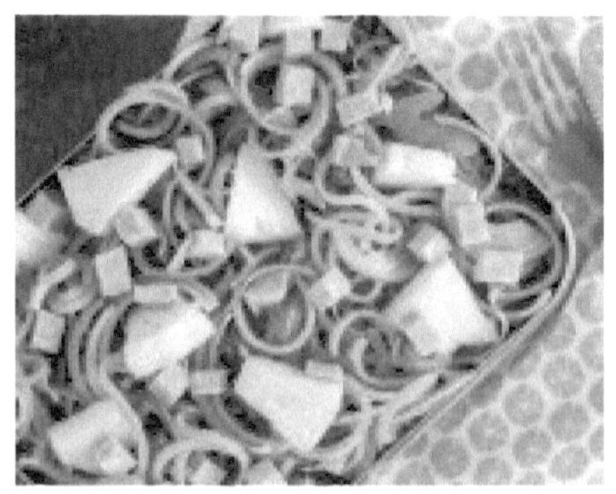

Preparation time: 10 minutes

Cooking time: 15 minutes

Servings: 1

Ingredients:

1 hand Arugula

1/2 pieces Red onion

1 piece winter carrot

2 pieces Pineapple slices

80 g Diced ham

1 pinch Salt

1 pinch Black pepper

Directions:

Cut the red onion into thin half rings.

Remove the peel and hard core from the pineapple and cut the pulp into thin pieces.

Clean the carrot and use a spiralizer to make strings.

Mix rocket and carrot in a bowl. Spread this over a plate.

Spread the red onion, pineapple and diced ham over the rocket.

Drizzle olive oil and balsamic vinegar on the salad to your taste.

Season it with salt and pepper.

Nutrition:

Calories: 150

Total Fat: 2.8 g

Cholesterol: 2 mg

Sodium: 42 mg

Potassium: 172 mg

Carbohydrates: 23 g

Protein: 2 g

Fresh Salad with Orange Dressing

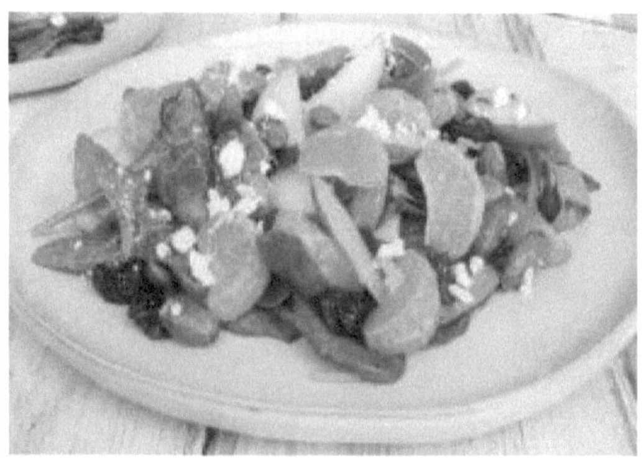

Preparation time: 10 minutes

Cooking time: 15 minutes

Servings: 1

Ingredients:

1 / 2 fruit Salad

1 piece yellow bell pepper

1 piece Red pepper

100 g Carrot (grated)

1 hand Almonds

Dressing:

4 tablespoon Olive oil

110 ml Orange juice (fresh)

1 tablespoon Apple cider vinegar

Directions:

Clean the peppers and cut them into long thin strips.

Tear off the lettuce leaves and cut them into smaller pieces.

Mix the salad with the peppers and the carrots processed in a bowl.

Roughly chop the almonds and sprinkle over the salad.

Mix all the ingredients for the dressing in a bowl.

Pour the dressing over the salad just before serving.

Nutrition:

Calories: 46.6

Total Fat: 0.1 g

Sodium: 230.8 mg

Potassium: 35.6 mg

Total Carbohydrates: 5.6 g

Protein: 0.7 g

Sweet Potato Hash Brown

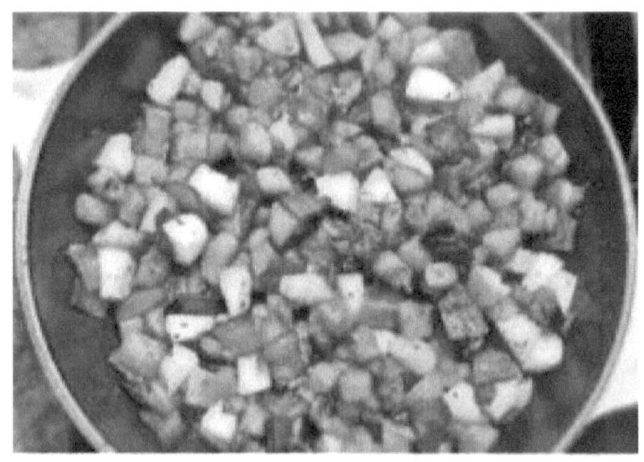

Preparation time: 5 minutes

Cooking time: 15 minutes

Servings: 2

Ingredients:

1 pinch Celtic sea salt

1 tablespoon Coconut oil

2 pieces Sweet potato

2 pieces Red onion

2 teaspoons Balsamic vinegar

1 piece Apple

125 g lean bacon strips

Directions:

Clean the red onions and cut them into half rings.

Heat a pan with a little coconut oil over medium heat. Fry the onion until it's almost done.

Add the balsamic vinegar and a pinch of salt and cook until the balsamic vinegar has boiled down. Put aside.

Peel the sweet potatoes and cut them into approx. 1.5 cm cubes.

Heat the coconut oil in a pan and fry the sweet potato cubes for 10 minutes.

Add the bacon strips for the last 2 minutes and fry them until you're done.

Cut the apple into cubes and add to the sweet potato cubes. Let it roast for a few minutes.

Then add the red onion and stir well.

Spread the sweet potato hash browns on 2 plates.

Nutrition:

Calories: 101

Total Fat: 7 g

Sodium: 5 mg

Potassium: 97 mg

Carbohydrates: 9 g

Protein: 0.8 g

Herby French Fries with Herbs and Avocado Dip

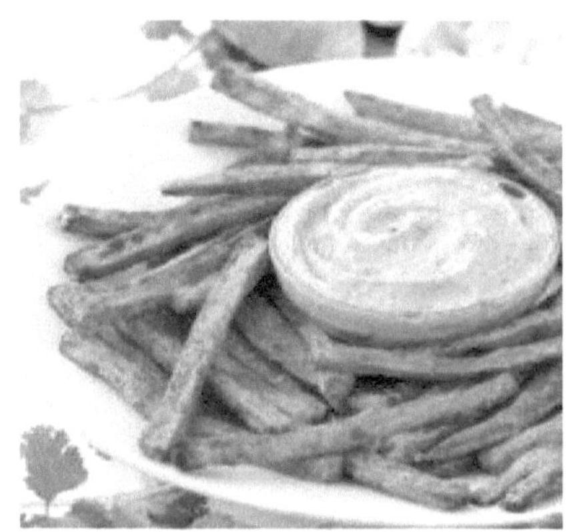

Preparation time: 15 minutes

Cooking time: 35 minutes

Servings: 1

Ingredient:

For the Fries:

1/2 pieces Celery

150 g Sweet potato

1 teaspoon dried oregano

1 / 2 teaspoon Dried basil

1/2 teaspoon Celtic sea salt

1 teaspoon Black pepper

1 1/2 tablespoon Coconut oil (melted)

Baking paper sheet

For the avocado dip:

1 piece Avocado

4 tablespoons Olive oil

1 tablespoon Mustard

1 teaspoon Apple cider vinegar

1 tablespoon Honey

2 cloves Garlic (pressed)

1 teaspoon dried oregano

Directions:

Preheat the oven to 205 ° C.

Peel the celery and sweet potatoes.

Cut the celery and sweet potatoes into (thin) French fries.

Place the French fries in a large bowl and mix with the
coconut oil and herbs.

Shake the bowl a few times so that the fries are covered
with a layer of the oil and herb mixture.

Place the chips in a layer on a baking sheet lined with
baking paper or on a grill rack.

Bake for 25-35 minutes (turn over after half the time) until
they have a nice golden brown color and are crispy.

For the avocado dip:

Puree all ingredients evenly with a hand blender or blender.

Nutrition:

Calories: 459

Total Fat: 27 g

Total Carbohydrates: 50 g

Protein: 4 g

Spiced Burger

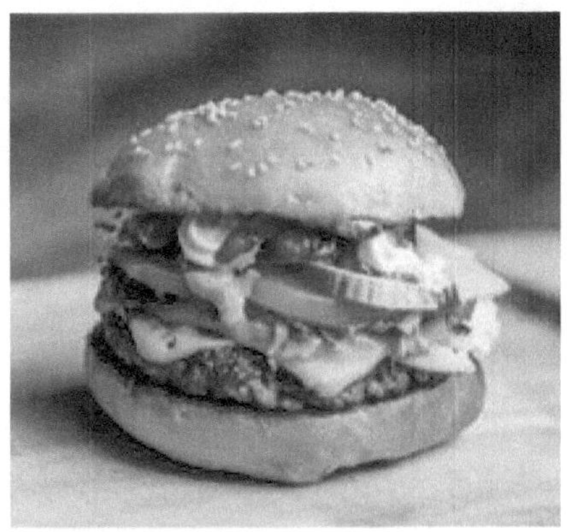

Preparation time: 20 minutes

Cooking time: 30 minutes

Serving: 1

Ingredients:

Ground beef 250 g

1 clove Garlic

1 teaspoon dried oregano

1 teaspoon Paprika powder

1 / 2 tsp. Caraway ground

Ingredients toppings:

4 pieces Mushrooms

1 piece Little Gem

1/4 pieces Zucchini

1/2 pieces Red onion

1 piece Tomato

Directions:

Squeeze the clove of garlic.

Mix all the ingredients for the burgers in a bowl. Divide the mixture into two halves and crush the halves into hamburgers.

Place the burgers on a plate and put in the fridge for a while.

Cut the zucchini diagonally into 1 cm slices.

Cut the red onion into half rings. Cut the tomato into thin slices and cut the leaves of the Little Gem salad.

Grill the hamburgers on the grill until they're done.

Place the mushrooms next to the burgers and grill on both sides until cooked but firm.

Place the zucchini slices next to it and grill briefly.

Now it's time to build the burger: Place 2 mushrooms on a plate then stack the lettuce, a few slices of zucchini and tomatoes. Then put the burger on top and finally add the red onion.

Nutrition:

Calories: 158

Fat: 8 g

Total Carbohydrates: 17 g

Protein: 3 g

Ganache Squares

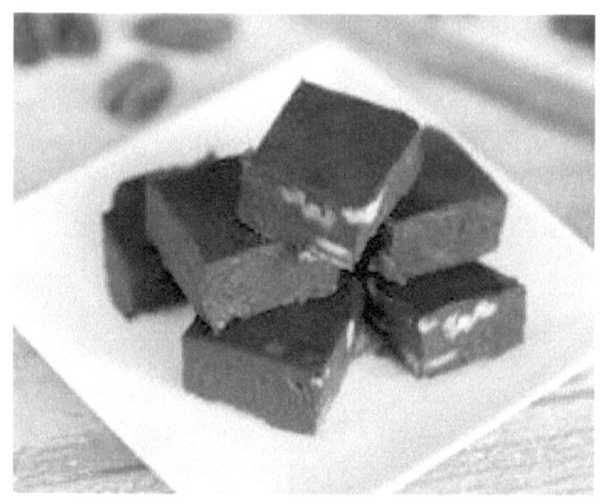

Preparation time: 15 minutes

Cooking time: 2 hours and 20 minutes

Servings: 10

Ingredients:

250 ml Coconut milk (can)

1 1/2 tablespoon Coconut oil

100 g Honey

1/2 teaspoon Vanilla extract

350 g pure chocolate (70% cocoa)

1 pinch Salt

2 hands Pecans

Directions:

Place the coconut milk in a saucepan and heat for 5 minutes over medium heat.

Add the vanilla extract, coconut oil and honey and cook for 15 minutes. Add a pinch of salt and stir well.

Break the chocolate into a bowl and pour the hot coconut milk over it. Keep stirring until all of the chocolate has dissolved in the coconut milk.

In the meantime, roughly chop the pecans. Heat a pan without oil and roast the pecans.

Stir the pecans through the ganache.

Let the ganache cool to room temperature. (You may be able to speed this up by placing the bowl in a bowl of cold water.)

Line a baking tin with a sheet of parchment paper. Pour the cooled ganache into it.

Place the ganache in the refrigerator for 2 hours to allow it to harden.

When the ganache has hardened, you can take it out of the mold and cut it into the desired shape.

Nutrition:

Calories: 141

Fat: 11 g

Carbohydrates: 9 g

Protein: 1 g

Date Candy

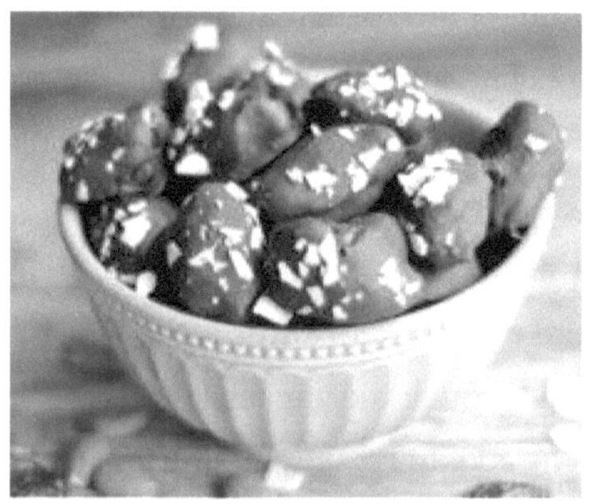

Preparation time: 20 minutes

Cooking time: 3 – 4 hours

Servings: 10

Ingredients:

10 pieces Medjool dates

1 hand Almonds

100 g pure chocolate (70% cocoa)

2 1/2 tablespoon Grated coconut

Directions:

Melt chocolate in a water bath.

Roughly chop the almonds.

In the meantime, cut the dates lengthways and take out the core.

Fill the resulting cavity with the roughly chopped almonds and close the dates again.

Place the dates on a sheet of parchment paper and pour the melted chocolate over each date.

Sprinkle the grated coconut over the chocolate dates.

Place the dates in the fridge so the chocolate can harden.

Nutrition:

100% joy!

Paleo Bars with Dates and Nuts

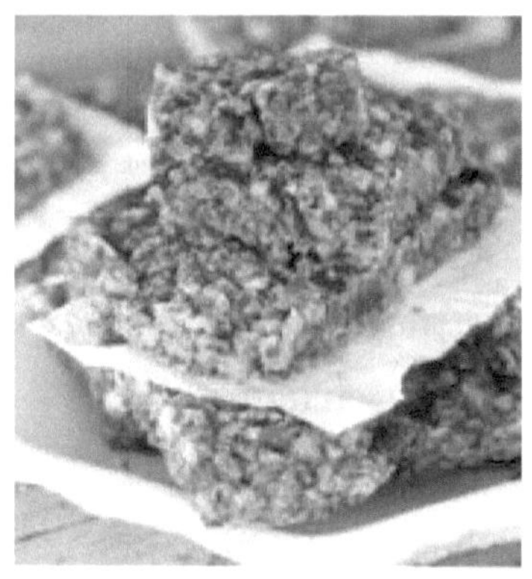

Preparation time: 10 minutes

Cooking time: 15 minutes

Servings: 16

Ingredients:

180 g Dates

60 g Almonds

60 g Walnuts

50 g Grated coconut

1 teaspoon Cinnamon

Directions:

Roughly chop the dates and soak them in warm water for 15 minutes.

In the meantime, roughly chop the almonds and walnuts.

Drain the dates.

Place the dates with the nuts, coconut and cinnamon in the food processor and mix to an even mass. (But not too long, crispy pieces or nuts make it particularly tasty)

Roll out the mass on 2 baking trays to form an approximately 1 cm thick rectangle.

Cut the rectangle into bars and keep each bar in a piece of parchment paper.

Nutrition:

Calories: 227

Total Fat: 19 g

Sodium: 9 mg

Carbohydrates: 12 g

Protein: 5 g

Hazelnut Balls

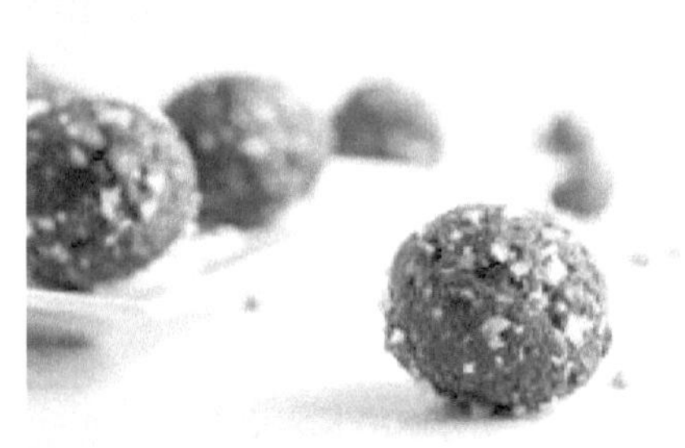

Preparation time: 20 minutes

Cooking time: 4 – 5 hours

Servings: 10

Ingredients:

130 g Dates

140 g Hazelnuts

2 tablespoon Cocoa powder

1/2 teaspoon Vanilla extract

1 teaspoon Honey

Directions:

Put the hazelnuts in a food processor and grind them until
you get hazelnut flour (you can also use ready-made
hazelnut flour).
Put the hazelnut flour in a bowl and set aside.
Put the dates in the food processor and grind them until
you get a ball.
Add the hazelnut flour, vanilla extract, cocoa and honey
and pulse until you get a nice and even mix.
Remove the mixture from the food processor and turn it
into beautiful balls.
Store the balls in the fridge.

Nutrition:

Calories: 73
Total Fat: 5 g
Total Carbohydrates: 5 g
Protein: 1 g

Pine and Sunflower Seed Rolls

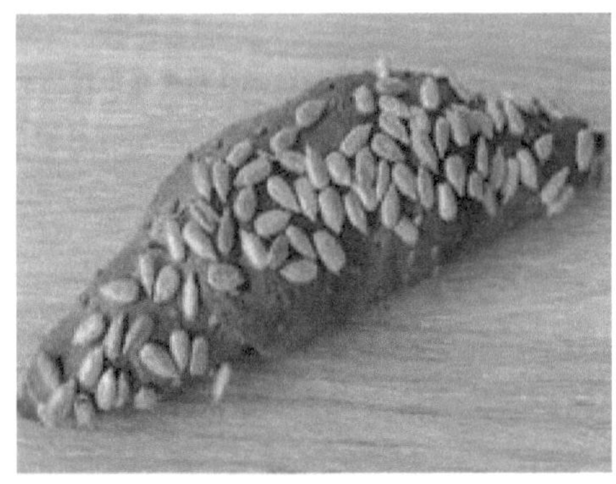

Preparation time: 20 minutes

Cooking time: 35 minutes

Servings: 10

Ingredients:

120 g Tapioca flour

1 teaspoon Celtic sea salt

4 tablespoon Coconut flour

120 ml Olive oil

120 ml Water (warm)

1 piece Egg (beaten)

150 g Pine nuts (roasted)

150 g Sunflower seeds (roasted)

Baking paper sheet

Directions:

Preheat the oven to 160 ° C.

Put the pine nuts and sunflower seeds in a small bowl and set aside.

Mix the tapioca with the salt and tablespoons of coconut flour in a large bowl. Pour the olive oil and warm water into the mixture.

Add the egg and mix until you get an even texture. If the dough is too thin, add 1 tablespoon of coconut flour at a time until it has the desired consistency.

Wait a few minutes between each addition of the flour so that it can absorb the moisture. The dough should be soft and sticky.

With a wet tablespoon, take tablespoons of batter to make a roll. Put some tapioca flour on your hands so the dough doesn't stick. Fold the dough with your fingertips instead of rolling it in your palms.

Place the roll in the bowl of pine nuts and sunflower seeds and roll it around until covered.

Line a baking sheet with parchment paper. Place the buns on the baking sheet.

Bake in the preheated oven for 35 minutes and serve warm.

Nutrition:

Calories: 163

Total Fat: 14 g

Fiber: 3 g

Total Carbohydrates: 6.5 g

Protein: 5 g

Banana Dessert

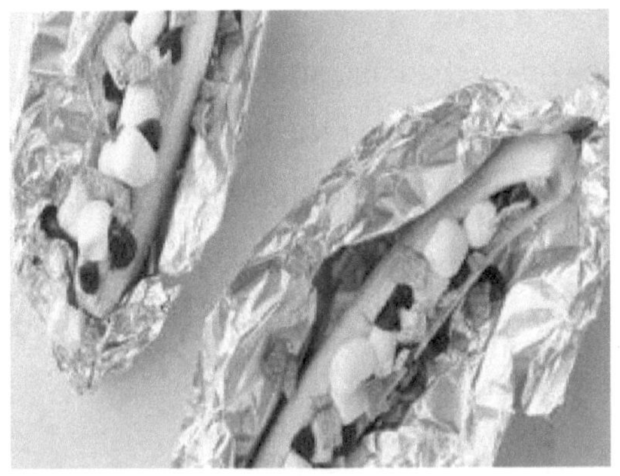

Preparation time: 5 minutes

Cooking time: 4 minutes

Servings: 2

Ingredients:

2 pieces Banana (ripe)

2 tablespoons pure chocolate (70% cocoa)

2 tablespoons Almond leaves

Directions:

Chop the chocolate finely, cut the banana lengthwise, but not completely, as the banana must serve as a casing for the chocolate.

Slightly slide on the banana, spread the finely chopped chocolate and almonds over the bananas.

Fold a kind of boat out of the aluminum foil that supports the banana well, with the cut in the banana facing up.

Place the two packets and grill them for about 4 minutes until the skin is dark.

Nutrition:

Calories: 105

Total Fat: 0.4 g

Sodium: 1.2 mg

Total Carbohydrates: 27 g

Protein: 1.3 g

Fiber: 3 g

Strawberry Popsicles with Chocolate Dip

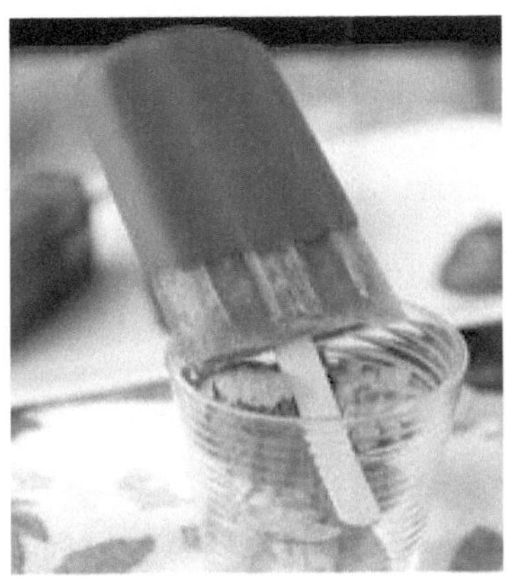

Preparation time: 20 minutes

Cooking time: 5 – 6 hours

Servings: 4

Ingredients:

125 g Strawberries

80 ml Water

100 g pure chocolate (70% cocoa)

Directions:

Clean the strawberries and cut them into pieces. Puree the strawberries with the water.

Pour the mixture into the Popsicle mold and put it in a skewer.

Place the molds in the freezer so the popsicles can freeze hard.

Once the popsicles are frozen hard, you can melt the chocolate in a water bath.

Dip the popsicles in the melted chocolate mixture.

Nutrition:

Calories: 60

Fiber: 1 g

Sugars: 14 g

Total Carbohydrates: 15 g

Strawberry and Coconut Ice Cream

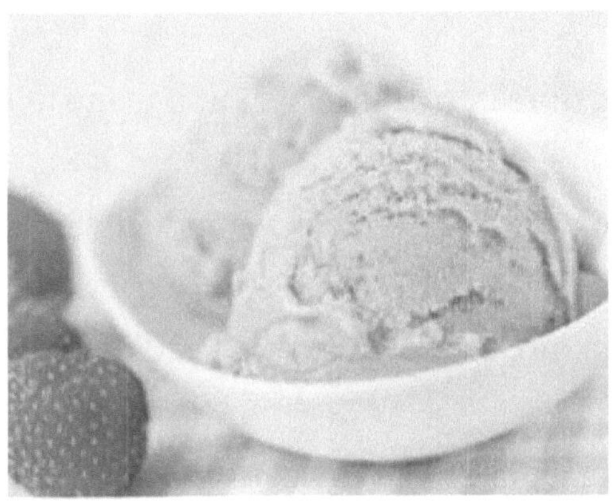

Preparation time: 20 minutes

Cooking time: 1 hour

Servings: 1

Ingredients:

400 ml Coconut milk (can)

1 hand Strawberries

1/2 pieces Lime

3 tablespoons Honey

Directions:

Clean the strawberries and cut them into large pieces.

Grate the lime, 1 teaspoon of lime peel is required. Squeeze the lime.

Put all ingredients in a blender and puree everything evenly.

Pour the mixture into a bowl and put it in the freezer for 1 hour.

Take the mixture out of the freezer and put it in the blender. Mix them well again.

Pour the mixture back into the bowl and freeze it until it is hard.

Before serving; take it out of the freezer about 10 minutes before scooping out the balls.

Nutrition:

Calories: 200

Total Fat: 11 g

Cholesterol: 0 mg

Sodium: 5 mg

Total Carbohydrates: 23 g

Protein: 1 g

Coffee Ice Cream

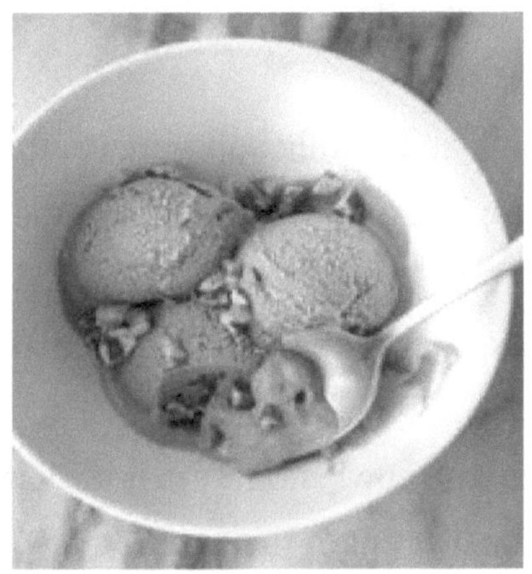

Preparation time: 15 minutes

Cooking time: 1 hour

Servings: 1

Ingredients:

180 ml Coffee

8 pieces Medjool dates

400 ml Coconut milk (can)

1 teaspoon Vanilla extract

Directions:

Make sure that the coffee has cooled down before using it.

Cut the dates into rough pieces.

Place the dates and coffee in a food processor and mix to an even mass.

Add coconut milk and vanilla and puree evenly.

Pour the mixture into a bowl and put it in the freezer for 1 hour.

Take the mixture out of the freezer and scoop it into the blender.

Pour it back into the bowl and freeze it until it's hard.

When serving; take it out of the freezer a few minutes before scooping ice cream balls with a spoon.

Nutrition:

Calories: 140

Total Fat: 7 g

Cholesterol: 25 mg

Sodium: 35 mg

Carbohydrates: 16 g

Banana Strawberry Milkshake

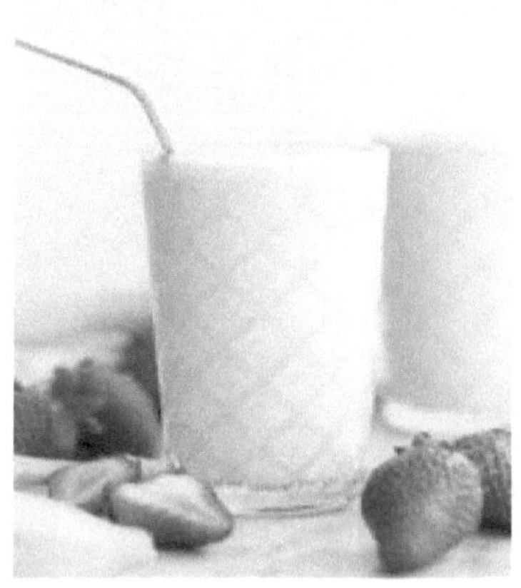

Preparation time: 10 minutes

Cooking time: 10 minutes

Servings: 1

Ingredients:

2 pieces Banana (frozen)

1 hand Strawberries (frozen)

250 ml Coconut milk (can)

Directions:

Peel the bananas, slice them and place them in a bag or on a tray. Put them in the freezer the night before.

Put all ingredients in the blender and mix to an even milkshake.

Spread on the glasses.

Nutrition:

Calories: 110

Total Fat: 1 g

Cholesterol: 5 mg

Sodium: 40 mg

Carbohydrates: 23 g

Sugar: 16 g

Protein: 4 g

Lime and Ginger Green Smoothie

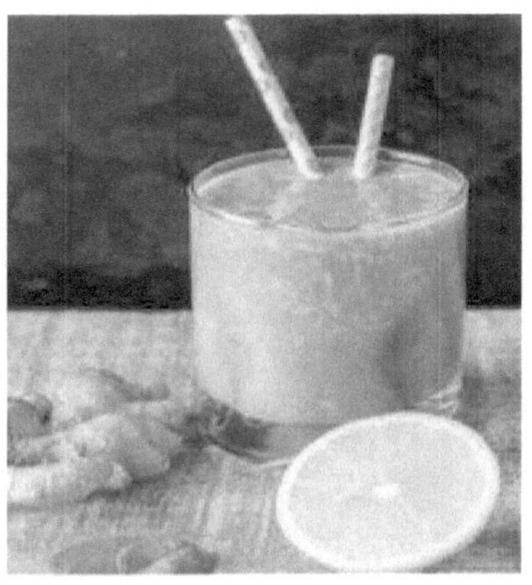

Preparation time: 5 minutes

Cooking time: 5 minutes

Servings: 1

Ingredients:

½ cup dairy free milk

½ cup water

½ teaspoon fresh ginger

½ cup mango chunks

Juice from 1 lime

1 tablespoon dried shredded coconut

1 tablespoon flaxseeds

1 cup spinach

Directions:

Blend together all the ingredients until smooth.
Serve and enjoy!

Nutrition:

Calories 178

Fat 1g

Carbohydrates 7g

Protein 4g

Turmeric Strawberry Green Smoothie

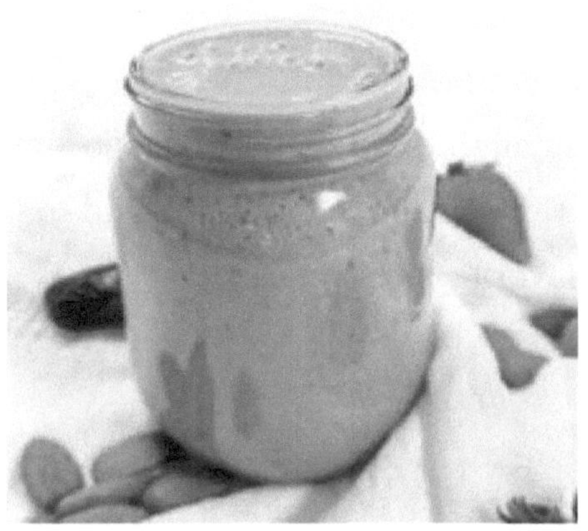

Preparation time: 5 minutes

Cooking time: 5 minutes

Servings: 1

Ingredients:

1 cup kale, stalks removed

1 teaspoon turmeric

1 cup strawberries

½ cup coconut yogurt

6 walnut halves

1 tablespoon raw cacao powder

1-2 mm slice of bird's eye chili

1 cup unsweetened almond milk

1 pitted Medjool date

Directions:

Blend together all the ingredients and enjoy immediately! Be careful how much almond milk you add so you can choose your favorite consistency.

Nutrition:

Calories 180

Fat 2.2g

Carbohydrates 12g

Protein 4g

Sirtfood Wonder Smoothie

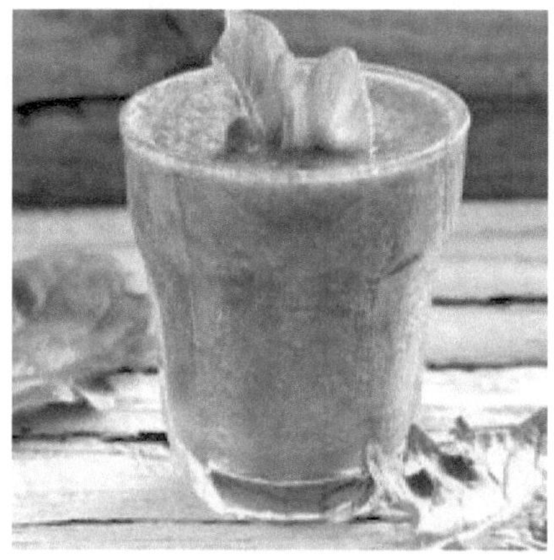

Preparation time: 5 minutes

Cooking time: 10 minutes

Servings: 1

Ingredients:

1 cup arugula (rocket)

2 cups organic strawberries or blueberries

1 cup kale

½ teaspoon matcha green tea

Juice of ½ lemon or lime

3 sprigs of parsley

½ cup of watercress

¾ cup of water

Directions:

Add all the ingredients except matcha to a blender and whizz up until very smooth.

Add the matcha green tea powder and give it a final blitz until well mixed.

Nutrition:

Calories 145

Fat 2g

Carbohydrates 7g

Protein 3g

Strawberry Spinach Smoothie

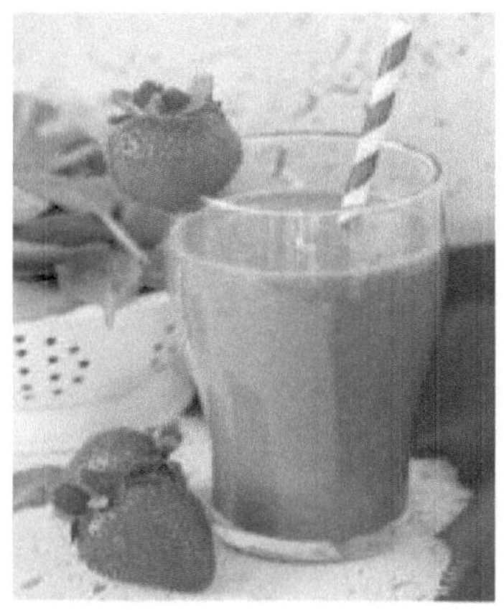

Preparation time: 5 minutes

Cooking time: 5 minutes

Servings: 1

Ingredients:

1 cup whole frozen strawberries

3 cups packed spinach

¼ cup frozen pineapple chunks

1 medium ripe banana, cut into chunks and frozen

1 cup unsweetened milk

1 tablespoon chia seeds

Directions:

Place all the ingredients in a high-powered blender.

Blend until smooth.

Enjoy!

Nutrition:

Calories 266

Fat 8g

Carbohydrates 48g

Protein 9g

Berry Turmeric Smoothie

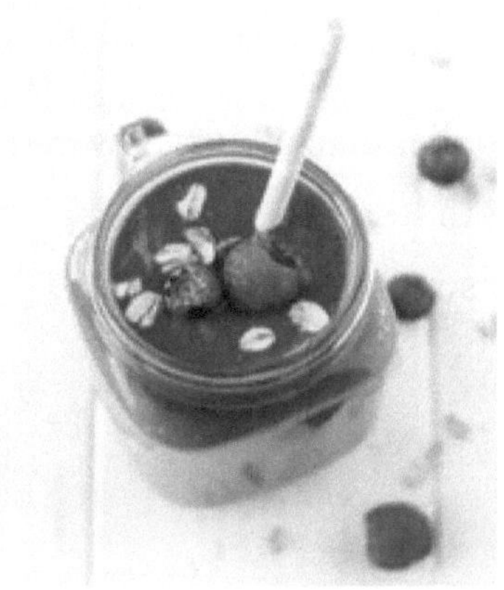

Preparation time: 5 minutes

Cooking time: 5 minutes

Servings: 1

Ingredients:

1 ½ cups frozen mixed berries (blueberries, blackberries and raspberries)

½ teaspoon ground turmeric

2 cups baby spinach

¾ cup unsweetened vanilla almond milk, or milk of choice

½ cup non-fat plain Greek yogurt, or yoghurt of choice

¼ teaspoon ground ginger

2-3 teaspoons honey

3 tablespoons old-fashioned rolled oats

Directions:

Place all the ingredients in a high-powered blender.

Blend until smooth.

Taste and adjust sweetness as desired.

Enjoy immediately!

Nutrition:

Calories 151

Fat 2g

Carbohydrates 27g

Protein 8g

Mango Green Smoothie

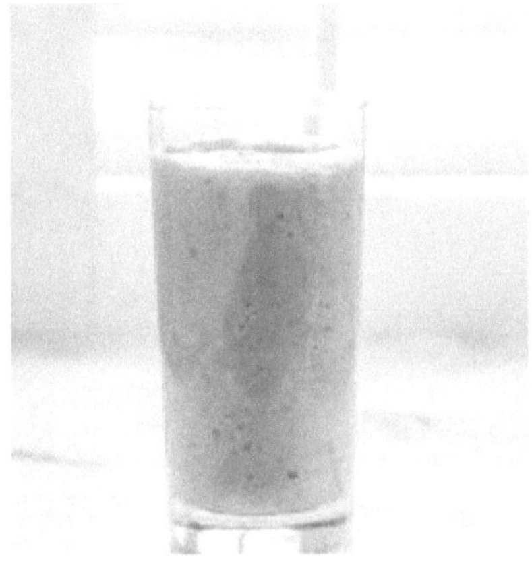

Preparation time: 3 minutes

Cooking time: 5 minutes

Servings: 1

Ingredients:

1 ½ cups frozen mango pieces

1 cup packed baby spinach leaves

1 ripe banana

¾ cup unsweetened vanilla almond milk

Directions:

Place all the ingredients in a blender.

Blend until smooth.

Enjoy!

Nutrition:

Calories 229

Fat 2g

Carbohydrates 72g

Protein 2g

Apple Avocado Smoothie

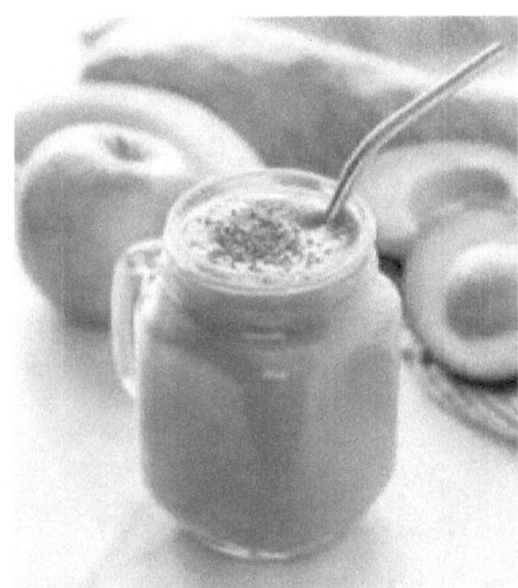

Preparation time: 5 minutes

Cooking time: 5 minutes

Servings: 1

Ingredients:

2 cups packed spinach

½ medium avocados

1 medium apple, peeled and quartered

½ medium bananas, cut into chunks and frozen

½ cup unsweetened almond milk

1 teaspoon honey

¼ teaspoon ground ginger
Small handful of ice cubes

Directions:

In the ordered list, add the almond milk, spinach, avocado, banana, apples, honey, ginger, and ice to a high-powered blender.
Blend until smooth.
Taste and adjust sweetness and spices as desired.
Enjoy immediately!

Nutrition:

Calories 206
Fat 11g
Carbohydrates 15g
Protein 5g

Kale Pineapple Smoothie

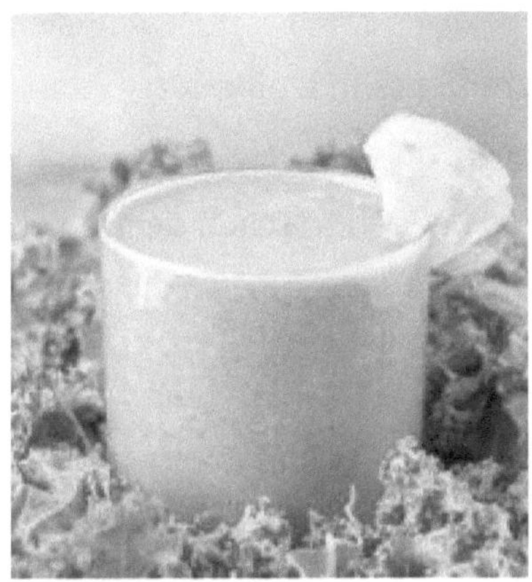

Preparation time: 5 minutes

Cooking time: 5 minutes

Servings: 1

Ingredients:

2 cups lightly packed chopped kale leaves, stems removed

¼ cup frozen pineapple pieces

1 frozen medium banana, cut into chunks

¼ cup non-fat Greek yogurt

2 teaspoons honey

¾ cup unsweetened vanilla almond milk, or any milk of choice

2 tablespoons peanut butter, creamy or crunchy

Directions:

Place all the ingredients in a blender.

Blend until smooth.

Add more milk as needed to reach desired consistency.

Enjoy immediately!

Nutrition:

Calories 187

Fat 9g

Carbohydrates 27g

Protein 8g

Blueberry Banana Avocado Smoothie

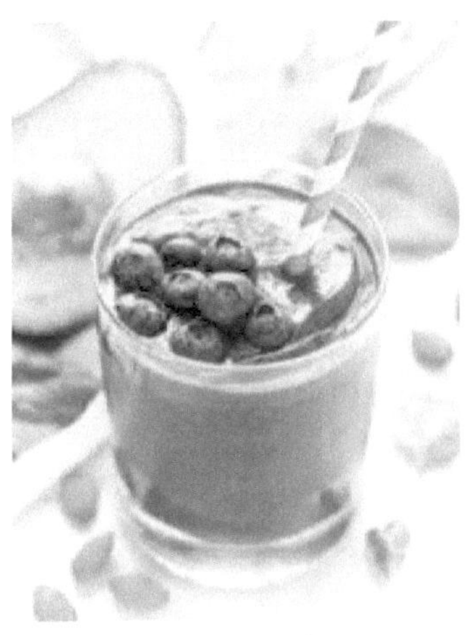

Preparation time: 10 minutes

Cooking time: 10 minutes

Servings: 1

Ingredients:

1 medium ripe banana, peeled

2 cups frozen blueberries

1 cup fresh spinach

1 tablespoon ground flaxseed meal

½ ripe avocados

1 tablespoon almond butter

¼ teaspoon cinnamon

½ cup unsweetened vanilla almond milk

Directions:

Place all the ingredients in your blender in the ordered list:
vanilla almond milk, spinach, banana, avocado,
blueberries, flaxseed meal, and almond butter.
Blend until smooth.
If you like a thicker smoothie, add a small handful of ice.
Enjoy immediately!

Nutrition:

Calories 298
Fat 14.4g
Carbohydrates 38.1g
Protein 8g

Carrot Smoothie

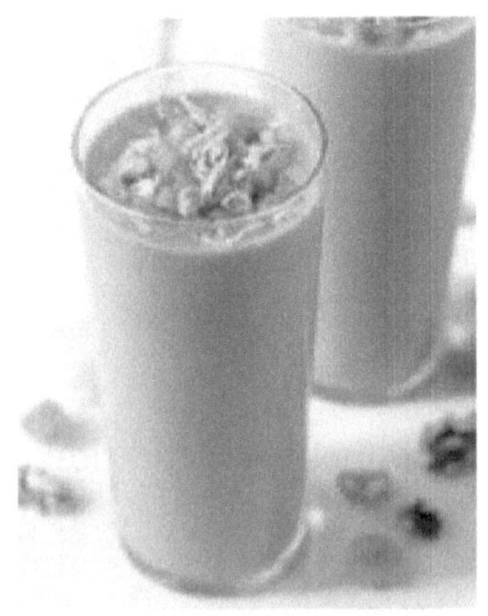

Preparation time: 10 minutes

Cooking time: 10 minutes

Servings: 1

Ingredients:

1 cup chopped carrots

¼ cup frozen diced pineapple

½ cup frozen sliced banana

¼ teaspoon cinnamon

1 tablespoon flaked coconut

½ cup Greek yogurt

2 tablespoons toasted walnuts

Pinch nutmeg

½ cup unsweetened vanilla almond milk, or milk of choice

For topping:

Shredded carrots, coconut, crushed walnuts

Directions:

Add all the ingredients into a blender.

Blend until smooth.

Enjoy immediately, topped with additional shredded carrots, coconut, and crushed walnuts as desired!

Nutrition:

Calories 279

Fat 6g

Carbohydrates 48g

Protein 7g

Matcha Berry Smoothie

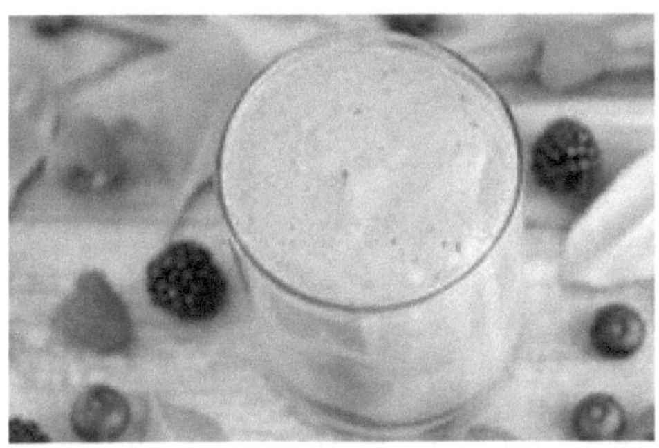

Preparation time: 5 minutes

Cooking time: 5 minutes

Servings: 1

Ingredients:

½ bananas

½-tablespoon matcha powder

1 cup almond milk

1 cup frozen blueberries

¼ teaspoon ground ginger

½ tablespoon chia seeds

¼ teaspoon ground cinnamon

Directions:

In a blender, blend the almond milk, banana, blueberries, matcha powder, chia seeds, cinnamon, and ginger until smooth.

Enjoy immediately!

Nutrition:

Calories 212

Fat 5g

Carbohydrates 34g

Protein 8g

Simple Grape Smoothie

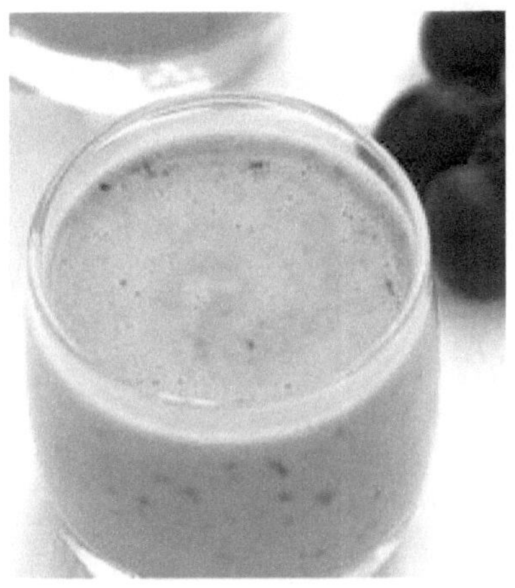

Preparation time: 5 minutes

Cooking time: 5 minutes

Servings: 1

Ingredients:

2 cups red seedless grapes

¼ cup grape juice

½ cup plain yogurt

1 cup ice

Directions:

Add grape juice to the blender. Then add yogurt and grapes. Add the ice last.
Blend until smooth and enjoy!

Nutrition:

Calories 161
Fat 4g
Carbohydrates 39g
Protein 2g

Ginger Plum Smoothie

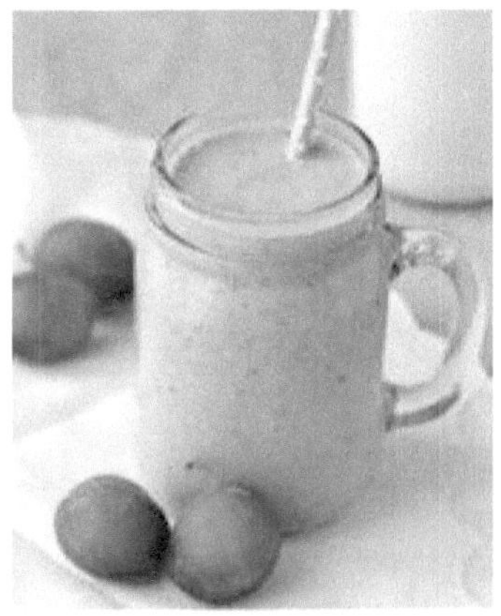

Preparation time: 5 minutes

Cooking time: 5 minutes

Servings: 1

Ingredients:

1 ripe plum, fresh or frozen, pitted but not peeled

½ cup plain yogurt

½ cup orange juice, or other fruit juice

1 teaspoon grated fresh ginger

Directions:

Put all the ingredients in a blender and blend until smooth.
Serve immediately and enjoy!

Nutrition:

Calories 124

Fat 2g

Carbohydrates 26g

Protein 3g

Kumquat Mango Smoothie

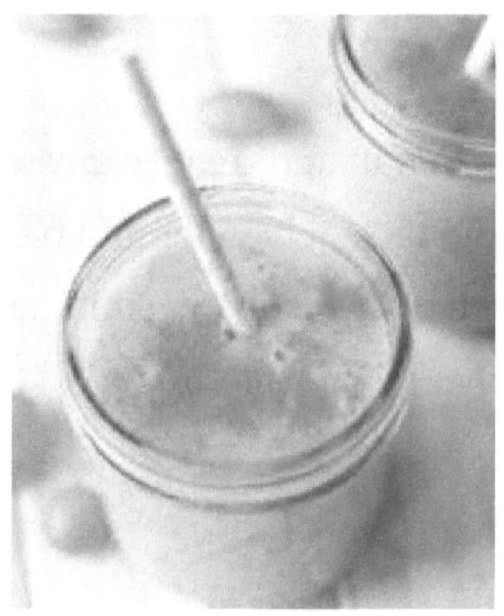

Preparation time: 10 minutes

Cooking time: 5 minutes

Servings: 1

Ingredients:

15 small kumquats

½ mango, peeled and chopped

¾ cup unsweetened almond milk

¼ teaspoon vanilla

½ cup plain yogurt

¼ teaspoon nutmeg

1 tablespoon honey

½ teaspoon ground cinnamon

5 ice cubes

Directions:

Cut the kumquats in half and remove any seeds.

Add all the ingredients to a blender and blend until smooth.

Garnish with another sprinkling of cinnamon, if desired.

Enjoy immediately!

Nutrition:

Calories 116

Fat 2g

Carbohydrates 22g

Protein 5g

Cranberry Smoothie

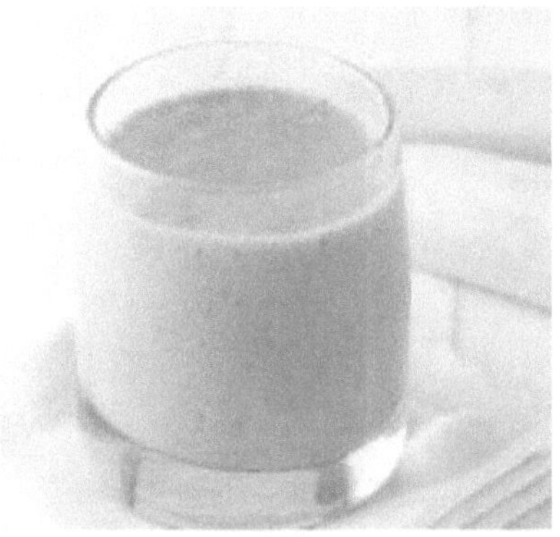

Preparation time: 5 minutes

Cooking time: 5 minutes

Servings: 1

Ingredients:

½ cup frozen cranberries

½ bananas

¼ cup orange juice

¼ cup frozen blueberries

¼ cup low fat Greek yogurt

Directions:

Add all the ingredients to a blender and blend until smooth.
Add a little more orange juice if you prefer it a little thinner.
Enjoy immediately!

Nutrition:

Calories 165

Fat 1g

Carbohydrates 31g

Protein 8g

Summer Berry Smoothie

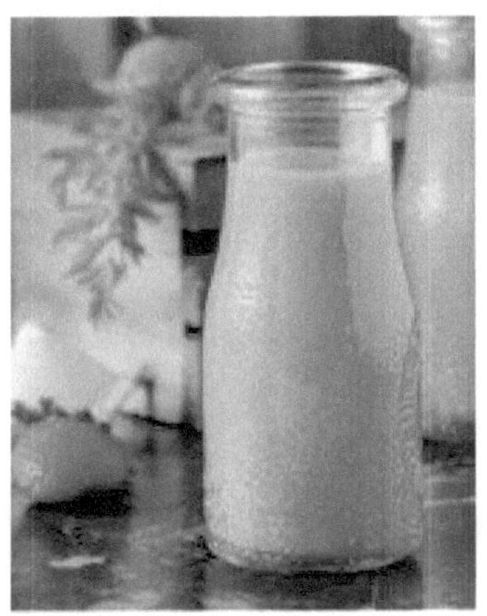

Preparation time: 10 minutes

Cooking time: 10 minutes

Servings: 1

Ingredients:

50g (2oz) blueberries

50g (2oz) strawberries

25g (1oz) blackcurrants

25g (1oz) red grapes

1 carrot, peeled

1 orange, peeled

Juice of 1 lime

Directions:

Place all of the ingredients into a blender and cover them with water. Blitz until smooth.

You can also add some crushed ice and a mint leaf to garnish.

Nutrition:

Calories: 110

Fat: 1 g

Carbohydrates: 20 g

Protein: 2 g

Mango, Celery and Ginger Smoothie

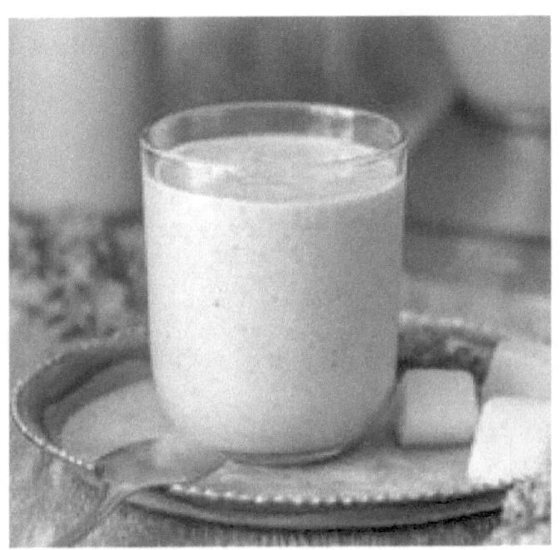

Preparation time: 10 minutes

Cooking time: 10 minutes

Servings: 1

Ingredients:

1 stalk of celery

50g (2oz) kale

1 apple, cored

50g (2oz) mango, peeled, de-stoned and chopped

2.5cm (1 inch) chunk of fresh ginger root, peeled and chopped

Directions:

Put all the ingredients into a blender with some water and blitz until smooth. Add ice to make your smoothie really refreshing.

Nutrition:

Calories: 92

Fat: 3 g

Carbohydrates: 22 g

Protein: 1 g

Orange, Carrot and Kale Smoothie

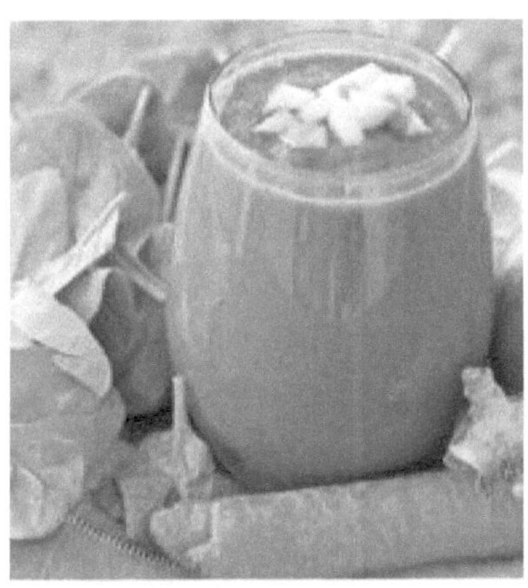

Preparation time: 5 minutes

Cooking time: 5 minutes

Servings: 1

Ingredients:

1 carrot, peeled

1 orange, peeled

1 stick of celery

1 apple, cored

50g (2oz) kale

½ teaspoon matcha powder

Directions:

Place all of the ingredients into a blender and add in enough water to cover them. Process until smooth, serve and enjoy.

Nutrition:

Calories: 150

Fat: 1 g

Carbohydrates: 36 g

Protein: 4 g

Creamy Strawberry and Cherry Smoothie

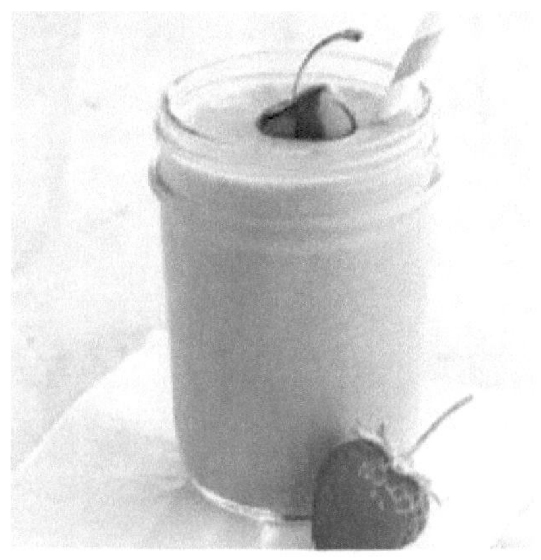

Preparation time: 5 minutes

Cooking time: 5 minutes

Servings: 1

Ingredients:

100g (3½ oz) strawberries

75g (3oz) frozen pitted cherries

1 tablespoon plain full-fat yogurt

175mls (6fl oz) unsweetened soya milk

Directions:

Place all of the ingredients into a blender and process until smooth. Serve and enjoy.

Nutrition:

Calories: 135

Fat: 1 g

Carbohydrates: 25 g

Protein: 3 g

Pineapple and Cucumber Smoothie

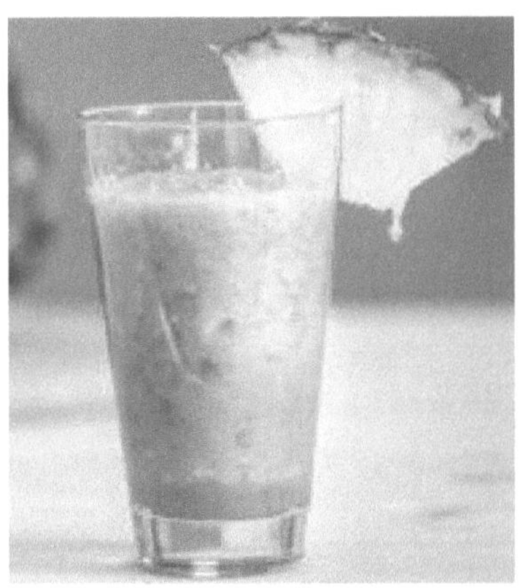

Preparation time: 5 minutes

Cooking time: 5 minutes

Servings: 1

Ingredients:

50g (2oz) cucumber

1 stalk of celery

2 slices of fresh pineapple

2 sprigs of parsley

½ teaspoon matcha powder

Squeeze of lemon juice

Directions:

Place all of the ingredients into blender with enough water to cover them and blitz until smooth.

Nutrition:

Calories: 125

Fat: 1 g

Carbohydrates: 22 g

Protein: 2 g

Avocado, Celery and Pineapple Smoothie

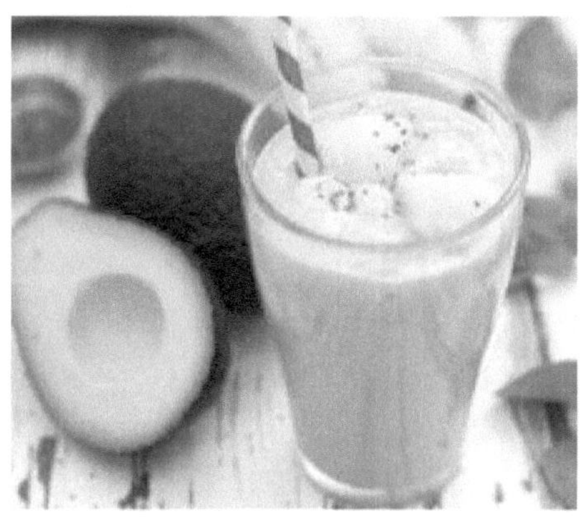

Preparation time: 5 minutes

Cooking time: 5 minutes

Servings: 1

Ingredients:

50g (2oz) fresh pineapple, peeled and chopped

3 stalks of celery

1 avocado, peeled & de-stoned

1 teaspoon fresh parsley

½ teaspoon matcha powder

Juice of ½ lemons

Directions:

Place all of the ingredients into a blender and add enough water to cover them - process until creamy and smooth.

Nutrition:

Calories: 138

Fat: 2 g

Carbohydrates: 25 g

Protein: 5g

Mango and Rocket (Arugula) Smoothie

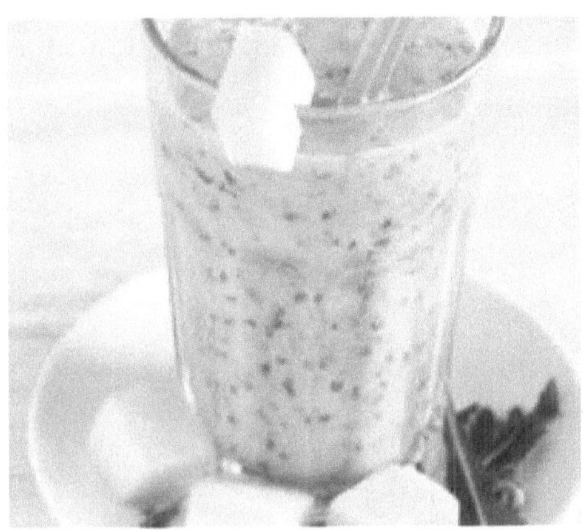

Preparation time: 5 minutes

Cooking time: 5 minutes

Servings: 1

Ingredients:

25g (1oz) fresh rocket (arugula)

150g (5oz) fresh mango, peeled, de-stoned and chopped

1 avocado, de-stoned and peeled

½ teaspoon matcha powder

Juice of 1 lime

Directions:

Place all of the ingredients into a blender with enough water to cover them and process until smooth. Add a few ice cubes and enjoy.

Nutrition:

Calories: 145

Fat: 2 g

Carbohydrates: 21 g

Protein: 5 g

Strawberry and Citrus Blend

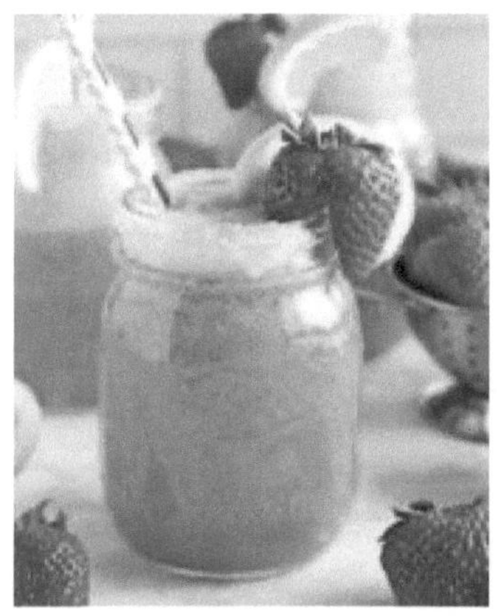

Preparation time: 5 minutes

Cooking time: 5 minutes

Servings: 1

Ingredients:

75g (3oz) strawberries

1 apple, cored

1 orange, peeled

½ avocado, peeled and de-stoned

½ teaspoon matcha powder

Juice of 1 lime

Directions:

Place all of the ingredients into a blender with enough water to cover them and process until smooth. Add ice to make it really refreshing.

Nutrition:

Calories: 112

Fat: 2 g

Carbohydrates: 23 g

Protein: 1 g

Orange and Celery Crush

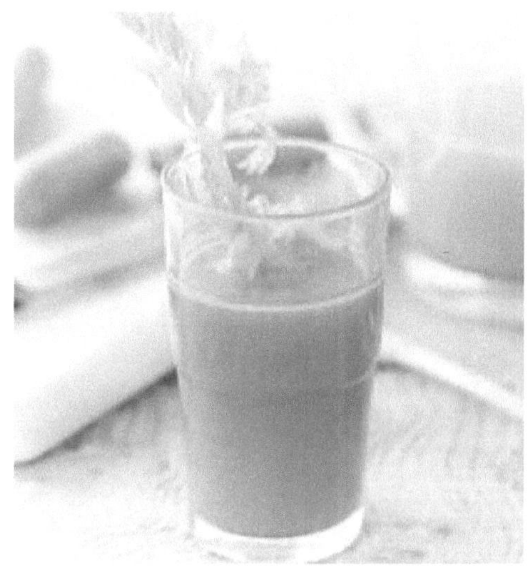

Preparation time: 5 minutes

Cooking time: 5 minutes

Servings: 1

Ingredients:

1 carrot, peeled

3 stalks of celery

1 orange, peeled

½ teaspoon matcha powder

Juice of 1 lime

Directions:

Place all of the ingredients into a blender with enough water to cover them and blitz until smooth. Add crushed ice to make your smoothie really refreshing.

Nutrition:

Calories: 180

Fat: 2 g

Carbohydrates: 25 g

Protein: 3 g

Chocolate, Strawberry and Coconut Crush

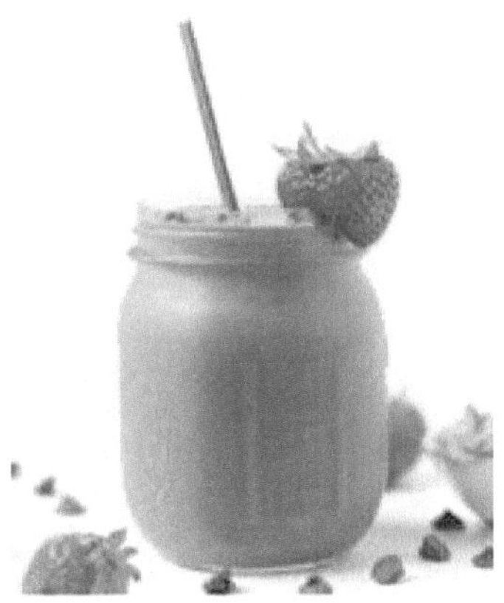

Preparation time: 5 minutes

Cooking time: 5 minutes

Servings: 1

Ingredients:

100mls (3½fl oz) coconut milk

100g (3½oz) strawberries

1 banana

1 tablespoon 100% cocoa powder or cacao nibs

1 teaspoon matcha powder

Directions:

Toss all of the ingredients into a blender and process them to a creamy consistency.

Add a little extra water if you need to thin it a little. Add crushed ice to make your smoothie really refreshing.

Nutrition:

Calories: 220

Fat: 3 g

Carbohydrates: 30 g

Protein: 5 g

Banana and Kale Smoothie

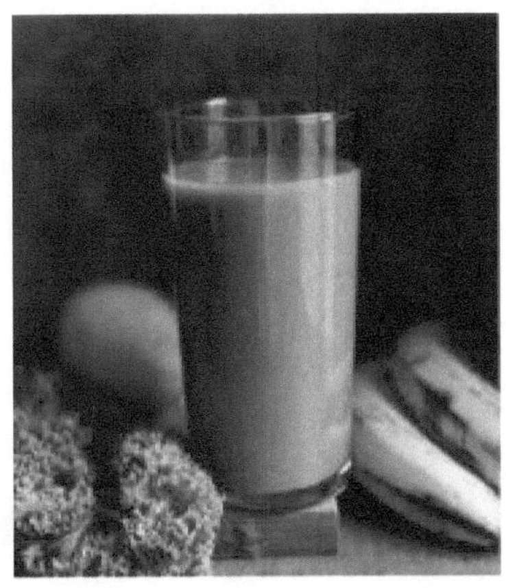

Preparation time: 5 minutes

Cooking time: 5 minutes

Servings: 1

Ingredients:

50g (2oz) kale

1 banana

200mls (7fl oz) unsweetened soya milk

Directions:

Place all of the ingredients into a blender with enough water to cover them and process until smooth. Add ice to make it really refreshing.

Nutrition:

Calories: 189

Fat: 2 g

Carbohydrates: 25 g

Protein: 3 g

Cranberry and Kale Crush

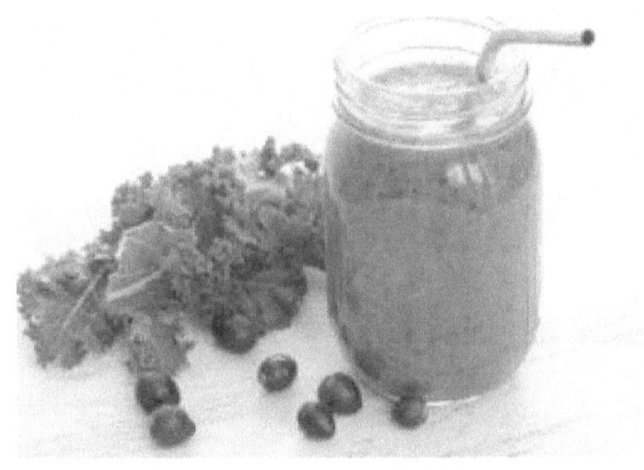

Preparation time: 5 minutes

Cooking time: 5 minutes

Servings: 1

Ingredients:

75g (3oz) strawberries

50g (2oz) kale

120mls (4fl oz) unsweetened cranberry juice

1 teaspoon chia seeds

½ teaspoon matcha powder

Directions:

Place all of the ingredients into a blender and process until smooth. Add some crushed ice and a mint leaf or two for a really refreshing drink.

Nutrition:

Calories: 213

Fat: 1 g

Carbohydrates: 28 g

Protein: 3 g

Grape, Celery and Parsley Reviver

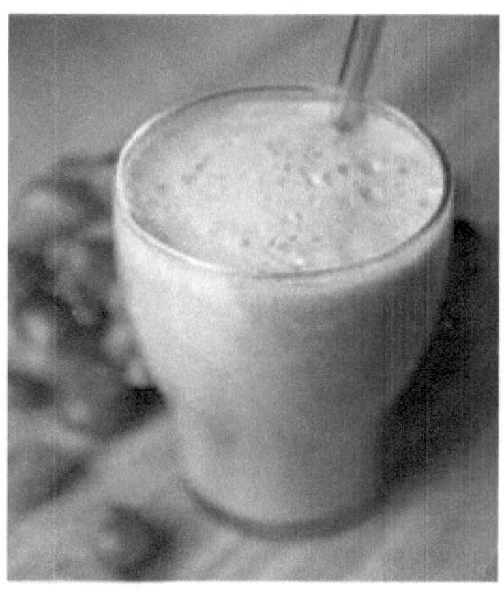

Preparation time: 5 minutes

Cooking time: 5 minutes

Servings: 1

Ingredients:

75g (3oz) red grapes

3 sticks of celery

1 avocado, de-stoned and peeled

1 tablespoon fresh parsley

½ teaspoon matcha powder

Directions:

Place all of the ingredients into a blender with enough water to cover them and blitz until smooth and creamy. Add crushed ice to make it even more refreshing.

Nutrition:

Calories: 253

Fat: 2 g

Carbohydrates: 35 g

Protein: 3 g

Grapefruit and Celery Blast

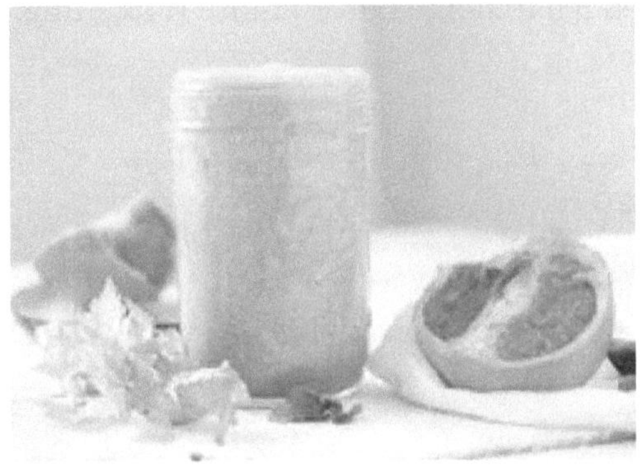

Preparation time: 5 minutes

Cooking time: 5 minutes

Servings: 1

Ingredients:

1 grapefruit, peeled

2 stalks of celery

50g (2oz) kale

½ teaspoon matcha powder

Directions:

Place all the ingredients into a blender with enough water to cover them and blitz until smooth.

Add crushed ice to make it even more refreshing.

Nutrition:

Calories: 220

Fat: 1 g

Carbohydrates: 31 g

Protein: 2 g

Tropical Chocolate Delight

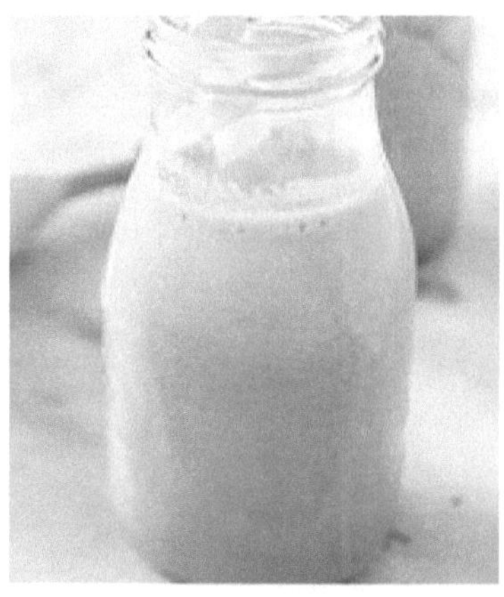

Preparation time: 5 minutes

Cooking time: 5 minutes

Servings: 1

Ingredients:

1 mango, peeled & de-stoned

75g (3oz) fresh pineapple, chopped

50g (2oz) kale

25g (1oz) rocket

1 tablespoon 100% cocoa powder or cacao nibs

150mls (5fl oz) coconut milk

Directions:

Place all of the ingredients into a blender and blitz until smooth. You can add a little water if it seems too thick. Add crushed ice to make it even more refreshing.

Nutrition:

Calories: 289

Fat: 4 g

Carbohydrates: 37 g

Protein: 3 g